# THE ROOTS OF BIOETHICS

# THE ROOTS OF BIOETHICS

HEALTH, PROGRESS, TECHNOLOGY, DEATH

DANIEL CALLAHAN

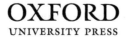
OXFORD
UNIVERSITY PRESS

# OXFORD
## UNIVERSITY PRESS

Oxford University Press is a department of the University of Oxford.
It furthers the University's objective of excellence in research, scholarship, and
education by publishing worldwide.

Oxford   New York

Auckland   Cape Town   Dar es Salaam   Hong Kong   Karachi
Kuala   Lumpur   Madrid   Melbourne   Mexico City   Nairobi
New Delhi   Shanghai   Taipei   Toronto

With offices in

Argentina   Austria   Brazil   Chile   Czech Republic   France   Greece
Guatemala   Hungary   Italy   Japan   Poland   Portugal   Singapore
South Korea   Switzerland   Thailand   Turkey   Ukraine   Vietnam

Oxford is a registered trademark of Oxford University Press in the UK
and certain other countries.

Published by Oxford University Press, Inc.
198 Madison Avenue, New York, New York 10016
www.oup.com

Library of Congress Cataloging-in-Publication Data
Callahan, Daniel, 1930–
The roots of bioethics : health, progress, technology, death/Daniel Callahan.
p. ; cm.
Includes bibliographical references.
ISBN 978-0-19-993137-8 (alk. paper)
I. Title.
[DNLM:   1. Bioethical Issues—Collected Works.   2. Bioethics—history—Collected Works.
3. Euthanasia—ethics—Collected Works.   4. Right to Die—ethics—Collected Works. WB 60]
174.2—dc23
2012008763

1  3  5  7  9  8  6  4  2

Printed in the United States of America
on acid-free paper

# CONTENTS

# ACKNOWLEDGMENTS

Chapter One. "The Hastings Center and the Early Years of Bioethics"
Publication Data. This was published in *The Kennedy Institute of Ethics Journal* (1999); 9.1: 53–71. © 1999 by The Johns Hopkins University Press.

Chapter Two. "A Memoir of an Interdisciplinary Career"
Publication Data. *Oxford Handbook of Interdisciplinary* (Oxford University Press 2010).

Chapter Three. "Minimalist Ethics"
Publication Data. *Hastings Center Report* (1981); 11 (5): 15–25. © 1981 The Hastings Center.

Chapter Four. "Individual good and Common Good"
Publication Data. This was first appeared in *Perspectives in Biology and Medicine*, 46.4 (2003); 496–507. Reprinted with permission by The Johns Hopkins University Press.

Chapter Five. "The WHO Definition of Health"
Publication Data. *Hastings Center Studies* (1973); 1 (3): 77–78. © 1973 The Hastings Center.

Chapter Six. "End-of-Life Care: A Philosophical or Management Problem?"
Publication Data. *The Journal of Law and Ethics* (Spring 2011); vol. 39 (2): 114–120. © 2012 John Wiley & Sons

Chapter Seven. "Death, Mourning, and Medical Progress"
Publication Data. This was published in *Perspectives in Biology and Medicine* 52.1 (2009); 103–115. © 2003 by The Johns Hopkins University Press.

Chapter Eight. "Terminating Life-Sustaining Treatment of the Demented"
Publication Data. *The Hastings Center Report* (1995): 25 (6): 25–31. © 1995 The Hastings Center

Chapter Nine. "Killing and Allowing to Die: Why It Is a Mistake to Derive an "Is" from an "Ought?" in Tonjorn Tannjorn, et. *Terminal Sedation: Euthanasia In Disguise* (Dordrecht: Kluwer, 2003).

Chapter Ten. "Rationing: Theory, Politics, and Passions"
Publication Date. *Hastings Center Report* (January-February 2011). © 2011 The Hastings Center.

Chapter Eleven. "Consumer-Directed health Care: Promise or Puffery?"
Publication Data. *Health Economics, Policy and Law*, vol. 3, issue 3 (July 2008): 301–311.

Chapter Twelve. "Societal Allocation of Resources for Patients with ESRD"
Publication Data. In Norman D. Levinsky, ed., *Ethics and the Kidney* (Oxford University
  Press, 2001): 201–211 © 2012. Oxford University Press

Chapter Thirteen. "Shaping Biomedical Research Priorities: The Case of the National
Institutes of Health"
Publication Data. *Health Care Analysis* (1997); 7. © 1999 Springer

Chapter Fourteen. "Time for a Change: Devising our Medical Future"
Publication Data: Unpublished manuscript

Chapter Fifteen. "Too Much of a Good Thing: How Splendid Technologies Can
Go Wrong"
Publication Data. *Hastings Center Report* (2003); 33 (2): 19–22. © 2003 The Hastings
  Center.

Chapter Sixteen. "Demythologizing the Stem Cell Juggernaut"
Publication Data. *Yale Journal of Health Politics, Law and Ethics* (2009); ix (2) (summer
  2012); 507–522. © 2012 Yale Journal of Health Politics, Law and Ethics.

Chapter Seventeen. "Health Technology Assessment Implementation: The
Politics of Ethics"
Publication Data. *Medical Decision Making* (January-February 2012); vol. 32 (1): E13–E19.
  © 2012 Sage Publications.

Chapter Eighteen. "Bioethics and Fatherhood"
Publication Data. *University of Utah Law Journal* (2002); (3): 735–46. © 2012 University
  of Utah.

# INTRODUCTION

## THE ROOTS OF BIOETHICS: HEALTH, PROGRESS, TECHNOLOGY, DEATH

I have had a long and happy life—good wife, good family, and good health—a life that also has been professionally satisfying. One can ask for nothing more. At age 82 I cannot expect life to get much better; that is not the usual trajectory of aging, as I am insistently reminded by my declining body. I am certainly pleased to have survived long enough to put together this collection of some of my articles over the years.

I have written many books and articles (and, of late, blogs) over the course of my career. I thoroughly need and enjoy writing. It is always a struggle to get things right, but for me a pleasurable kind of wrestling with oneself. Moreover, most scholars I know read, teach, and discuss a topic for many years and then cap off that effort with a book or articles, pulling things together. My way is just the opposite: I often take on topics I know little about in order to learn new things and to see where my research leads me. Half of the articles in this book were also written at the invitation of a journal editor or someone putting together a collection of papers. Often the request was to write about something of which I knew little. That made it irresistible to someone always looking for an occasion to write about something new, and someone who is hardly ever wise enough to say no. I do think those articles turned out as well as if I had thought up the topic myself.

The title of this collection of essays is meant to characterize the wide range of topics I have pursued over the years. Although trained as a philosopher, I have never had a great interest in ethical theories. They are still there in the back of my mind, but my starting point has been to begin with some basic categories of human life and medicine and to build up from there. The subtitle of this book catches four of them: (1) health (what it means to pursue health with a finite body); (2) progress (how we ought to evaluate progress, particularly medical progress); (3) technology (how we assess technologies for their human benefit); and (4) death (what should be the place of death in thinking about life and in understanding the goals of medicine). I might well have added "aging" (how medicine and policy should deal with the reality of aging societies) and "resource allocation" to that list (how we ought to fairly allocate scarce medical resources). The title of the book itself is meant to capture the importance of those basic categories for bioethics.

As explained more fully in one of the articles in this collection, I thoroughly enjoy interdisciplinary topics, requiring that one read widely, often about unfamiliar topics and in fields far removed from my own. I took great pleasure over the years in publishing articles in journals well outside the field of bioethics and ethics. Yet, there is a pitfall to publishing in such journals: one's colleagues may never see those articles. It is thus a special blessing to be able to reprint a number of those articles here, perhaps reaching the eyes of many who never heard of them.

The articles collected in this book are not only a good sampler of my writing but no less highlight the main themes of my work over many decades, particularly the last decade. There is considerable overlap among them, playing out similar melodies on a wide range of different instruments.

**Bioethics.** It seems fitting to start with bioethics, a field I had a hand in starting in 1969 with the founding of the Hastings Center. The first article, "*The Hastings Center and the Early Years of Bioethics*," tells that story, but with added commentary on the way the field of bioethics was shaping up. "*A Memoir of An Interdisciplinary Career*" highlights an important feature of the Hastings Center and my approach to bioethics. Although trained as a philosopher, I did not believe that philosophy should have a dominant role. Skepticism about the value of the reigning analytic philosophy of the day plus my wide humanities education in college, and the experiential complexity of many ethical issues, made obvious to me the need for a vigorous interplay of many fields.

The articles "*Minimalist Ethics*" and "*Individual Good and Common Good*," although published more than 20 years apart, could just as well have been published at the same time. Early on, I was unfriendly to the excessive dominance of the concept of autonomy in the emerging field and, as an alternative, was drawn to communitarianism as the antidote. I believed the hegemony of autonomy thinned the substance of ethics down to a brittle skeleton, demanding too little of us in our personal lives and insubstantial if given too much weight in policy decisions. Someone once called me an "autonomy basher," and that was a fair charge. Communitarianism is by no means a very precise notion, but it does offer a societal counterpoint to the individualism of autonomy.

**Aging, Death, and Medical Progress.** This topic covers a lot of territory, but to me sums up tightly interlocked issues. How should we think about aging and death in our individual and social lives, and where should the deep-seated value of medical progress in modern medicine fit into that kind of reflection? Medical progress has set its face against aging and death, treating them as enemies to be vanquished, setting no limits to that struggle, economic or otherwise. That kind of medicine, open-ended and never satisfied, seems to me a great mistake, and the articles in this section try to capture that conviction.

"*The WHO Definition of Health*" was my response to that much-publicized 1947 definition, which at face value seemed to put all human welfare and happiness under its aegis. That kind of breadth made little sense. Yet, as I thought further about it, I began to appreciate the definition. Applied carefully, it could offer some useful insights. I might have concluded long ago that the debate about it was over, but decided it is worth reprinting here after recently reading some enthusiastic support of the definition. "*End-of-Life Care: A Philosophical or Management Problem*" argues that it is a mistake to treat end-of-life decisions as solely a matter of better patient and physician education or an improvement of palliative care. On the contrary, those valuable goals need to be complemented by a consideration of death itself in our lives. There is remarkably little in the medical literature on death, and not much more in bioethics. What are we to make of the place of death in human life and in medicine? "*Death, Mourning, and Medical Progress*" makes in passing a similar point but looks more fully at the changing place of mourning in our society, not all of it good and, in its way, evading a confrontation with death.

"*Terminating Life-Sustaining Treatment of the Demented*" was a hard article to write, emotionally and philosophically. It is a peculiarly troubling issue. The rise in the number and proportion of the demented as the population ages and the baby boomers retire—with a projection of $1 trillion in costs by 2050 and some 50% of those older than 80 years likely to contract Alzheimer disease— makes it a major medical and familial problem. It is hard to find a baby boomer these days who has not had to cope with the dementia of at least one parent. The children of those boomers will in turn have the problem of caring for their parents. The essay *"Killing and Allowing to Die"* fits into this section because it looks at the question of whether there is any real ethical difference in turning off the respirator of a dying patient and directly killing the patient by a lethal injection. The late philosopher James Rachels made a strong and much-cited argument that there is no difference. Most doctors, I found, do not agree with him, and I was curious just why that is the case. I decided the doctors are right.

**Resource Allocation.** In 1987, I published *Setting Limits: Medical Goals In an Aging Society.* That was my first foray into the territory of resource allocation, in that case allocation to the elderly. The book received much attention, combined with sharp criticism for arguing that age itself would one day have to be used to set limits to expensive care. I also believed it necessary to examine what it means to grow old, and how that biologic inevitability should affect the way we think about resource allocation.

The first article in this section, *"Rationing: Theory, Passion, and Politics,"* was written as a response to the debate on controlling Medicare costs that broke out during the recent and rancorous health reform debate. My interest, however, focused on the ferocity of that debate and the way the word "rationing" became a lightning rod for ideologic struggles. Those of us in bioethics need to dive into the politics of that debate, moving away from the procedural generalities and unreal tidiness that mark a good deal of academic writing on just resource allocation. The article *"Consumer-Directed Health Care: Promise or Puffery"* was written in response to a request by a British healthcare journal to explain just what the American interest in that topic is all about. The politics of the concept interested me as much as its economic significance.

The *"Societal Allocation of Resources for Patients with ESRD"* was also written on request, one I was pleased to accept because ESRD has its own unique history in bioethics, going back to the famous 1960 Seattle committee that had to make terribly difficult decisions about who should gain access to kidney dialysis in the face of a great shortage of the then-new dialysis machine. *"Shaping Biomedical Research Priorities Priorities: The Case of the National Institutes of Health"* came about as an offshoot of a great international interest during the 1980s and 1990s in priority setting in healthcare systems. I wondered why there was no complementary interest in the setting of research priorities, and the NIH seemed a good place to look for an answer. So far as I know, this article is the only one to look at that topic in a systematic way, and I am surprised that others have not taken it up.

The final article in this section, "Time for a Change: Devising Our Medical Future," is the original manuscript for a paper that was used as the basis for an article authored jointly by Dr. Sherwin Nuland and myself published in June of 2011 in *The New Republic.* I liked the original article, written by myself alone, better than the heavily edited joint version—not because I dislike Dr. Nuland's share in the published article, but because the editors more or less muddled the original argument. It is an article that sums up a major thread running through my writings in recent years: that it is not just the healthcare system that needs reform, but no less the understanding of medicine that lies behind the system.

**Technology.** A persistent theme that runs through the history of bioethics since the 1960s is that of medical technology, from the dialysis crisis of that era right up to the emergence in the past few years of synthetic biology. It is a topic from which I cannot stay away. *"Too Much of a Good Thing: How Splendid Technologies Can Go Wrong"* takes its point of departure from my daily commute to work, noting an ever-present traffic jam and observing that the rise and dominance of the automobile in American life has many parallels with the dominance of technology in American health care. The fact of multimile traffic backups, making auto commuting one of the most unpleasant features of American life, is matched by medical technology's costly impact on health care, simultaneously benefiting but also wreaking economic havoc with millions of Americans. We can neither give up automobiles and medical technology nor find a way to give them a more sensible place in our national life.

*"Demythologizing the Stem Cell Juggernaut"* is my idiosyncratic response to the hoopla and inflated claims that went with the research on embryonic stem cells of the late 1990s. One claim was that the research could eventually save 150 million lives. What most caught my attention, however, was the way in which the public and professional debate set it up as a matter of balancing the claims made on behalf of the embryos that would be destroyed in the research against the many lives that could be saved by the research. But the odd feature of that balancing effort was that all of the attention was focused on the embryo, as if the moral status of the lives to be saved was so self-evidently beneficial that it needed no analysis or defense. I had previously made a case in my 2003 book, *What Price Better Health: Hazards of the Research Imperative*, that biomedical research is a human good, but not a moral obligation. My article used that argument to deflate the claims made on behalf of embryonic stem cell research.

The article on *"Health Technology Assessment"* came out of a panel I was on at a meeting of the Society for Medical Decision Making, a group I had never heard of when I accepted their invitation to prepare a paper on the ethical problems of decision making. I chose as a valuable case study the 2009 debate on the controversial American public health guidelines on mammography screening for breast cancer of women under the age of 50. Once again, I was drawn to the mix of ethics and interest group politics that was a prominent feature of that debate. It was in many ways a debate made all the more difficult by the way ethical values and principles could be used for partisan purposes.

The final article, "*Bioethics and Fatherhood*," written for a collection of papers on bioethics and the family, is an effort on my part to argue that sperm donations should not take place unless the donor is willing to bear the full burden of biologic fatherhood. A donor is a father and society and should not, by legal fiat, set aside that genetic link as if irrelevant, assigning the role of father to someone else. I was particularly curious why feminists—knowing all too well the feckless ways of men not wanting to take responsibility for children they procreate—let sperm donation get by under their radar. That was not a popular argument, but I was surprised some years later to receive letters from women who had been procreated with donated sperm and wanted either the right to know who the donor was or to have donations banned altogether. That was gratifying.

\* \* \* \* \* \* \*

I mention here that the MIT Press published in 2012 a memoir about my life and career, *In Search of The Good: A Life in Bioethics.* That book is an effort to better understand my own life and how that life expressed itself in starting the Hastings Center, and how my thinking about ethics developed over the years— not simply as an academic topic, but also as a way of conceiving and directing a particular kind of life.

# 1

## THE HASTINGS CENTER AND
## THE EARLY YEARS OF BIOETHICS

True beginnings are hard to discern. They are often little noticed at the time and in retrospect can sometimes be identified only in a more or less arbitrary way. So it is with the beginning of my own career in bioethics and the founding of the Hastings Center, both of which happened more or less simultaneously. Did they begin with my long childhood days in hospitals in the 1930s, the victim of a series of tenacious infections? Those were the pre-antibiotic days and the cures were far more painful than the infections. I was time and again carried kicking and screaming to the hospital. That sort of thing leaves a scar on one's psyche that is not readily erased, not to mention a life-long interest in medicine. Or did they begin with my interest in religion as an adolescent and in philosophy as a college student? Or was it when I became disillusioned with academic analytic philosophy as a graduate student and needed some other outlet for my intellectual thirsts? Or was it much later, when I began to see that bioethics was an emergent subject matter, suitable for a research center? I can't really answer those questions, and perhaps the proper metaphor is that of the origin of the Hudson River, not too far north of the Hastings Center: a cluster of small streams coming together until finally they make a river, leaving room for argument about just where exactly that happens.

What matters, though, is that there was a beginning and that now, 30 years later, my life in bioethics and the life of the Hastings Center go on. I find it most convenient to take up the story in the 1960s, when three streams converged to set the stage for bioethics in general and my entrance into it in particular. One of those streams was what we now think of as "the 60s," a time marked by assorted political and cultural upheavals and marked, in the case of medicine, by a sharp public and professional scrutiny of its institutions and practices. Medicine was opened for public inspection, not wholly of course but enough to be noticed. Another stream was marked by both a fear of and a fascination with the great technological changes medicine was creating. Those changes portended not simply new possibilities for health, such as raising the standards of what counts as good health; but also new ways of living a life, such as family planning and an extended and healthy old age. The third stream was a revolt in some branches of the humanities against the social isolation of the academy and a desire to let certain fields, especially philosophy, have some social bite, some "relevance" as the operative term of that era put it.

I will begin my story with the philosophy stream. I went to Yale as an undergraduate, mainly because I was a swimmer and that was the place to go in the 1940s and 1950s. But I was over the hill (or under the water) as a swimmer by my junior year and had to find something else to amuse me. That turned out to be an experimental interdisciplinary program, just right for someone who at that time had no specific career goals in mind but was drawn to the humanities. Only during my senior year did I decide I wanted to be a philosopher.

After three years in the army during the Korean War and an M.A. in philosophy from Georgetown–which I got at night while stationed in Washington–I entered the Harvard department of philosophy in the fall of 1956. It was anything but a congenial department. Of some 17 entering students in my year only three ever got their degrees; and my most famous classmates, Susan Sontag and the civil rights leader Bob Moses, were dropouts. The atmosphere was highly competitive, impersonal, utterly academic in the most narrow sense, and, worst of all, dominated by analytic philosophy, most of it imported from Oxford.

## MORAL PHILOSOPHY IN THE ANALYTIC MODE

Moral philosophy in that analytic mode focused almost entirely on the struggle between utilitarianism and deontology, but even that struggle was submerged beneath the even greater interest in metaethics, mired in the uses and status of moral concepts and language. Normative ethics was almost entirely absent. That kind of analytic ethics turned out to be tiresome, even deadly, fare for someone who had been drawn to philosophy by the example of Socrates, who asked large and annoying questions not in the academy but in the marketplace. Of that kind of ethics we heard little, just as we heard practically nothing of Aristotelian ethics. We were positively warned against existentialism and continental philosophy, which were dismissed as not philosophy at all.

What I did not realize at the time, hanging around the wrong circles I suppose, was that a number of other philosophers were reacting almost as negatively as I was. The founding of the journal *Philosophy and Public Affairs* in 1970 and the publication of John Rawls's book, *A Theory of Justice*, in 1971 signaled the beginning of a new era in moral and political philosophy. But that was not quite adequate for me. It soon became clear that most of the philosophers making that turn wanted to remain in the academy and saw their audience primarily as other philosophers, not doctors or lawyers, politicians or policymakers, and surely not the general public. It was a turn in any case too late for me. I wanted to get out of that world but, at the same time, find some meaningful and serious intellectual work.

As I drifted about in the 1960s, spending some time as a magazine editor (*Commonweal*) and a visiting professor here and there (Temple, Brown, and the University of Pennsylvania), I began stumbling across the biotechnological developments of that decade, truly a remarkable cascade: organ transplantation, prenatal diagnosis, respirators and ICUs, neonatal care, contraception and safe abortion, on and on. In 1967, I got interested in the problem of abortion, at a time when the abortion reform movement was agitating state legislatures. I began a book on that topic (Callahan 1970), which consumed some two full years of my time. In the process, while working in the splendid library of the New York Academy of Medicine and taking part in a few conferences, I became even more aware of the growing professional and public interest in ethics. It gradually occurred to me that here was a fertile area for a philosopher drawn to issues of practical ethics and no less drawn, from my undergraduate days, to interdisciplinary fields.

Apart from my abortion book, my first real taste of applied ethics came in 1968–1969, when I spent a year at the Population Council in New York, as a kind of resident ethicist. I was charged by its then-President, Bernard Berelson, to examine the ethical problems of family planning and population limitation programs. If I discovered there all the more how arresting and important ethical problems can be, I no less discovered how many professionals in many fields can be utterly indifferent to moral questions, something a little less true today. The reason for that indifference is not some moral hollowness, but instead the dominance of technical modes of thought and analysis and the lure of quantitative and scientific approaches to issues of biomedical practice and policy. Ethics appears, by contrast, woolly, indecisive, and impregnable to genuine progress. That is a false picture, but a persistent one in scientific and medical circles.

## ORGANIZING THE HASTINGS CENTER

At some point or other in 1968, I got the idea of starting a center in ethics. The issues were there, it appealed to my liking for applied ethics, and it seemed possible. But I had never started or run any kind of organization. "How do you do that?" I asked a variety of people. It's simple, they said, you get good people and a bit of money, give them an interesting idea to work with, and then spend 10 hours a day for 7 days a week single mindedly working out the nuts and bolts. The notion of a center had, moreover, some immediate plausibility: a number of articles and books were appearing on biomedical ethics, symposiums were being held and, time and again, the refrain was heard that "someone should be thinking about these problems."

The general advice I got was quite correct, and it just had to be carried out. My first and greatest break came when I presented my thinking about a center to a neighbor in Hastings-on-Hudson, Willard Gaylin, a psychiatrist, at a Christmas party in 1968. I had come to know Will over the previous few years as a lively and inquiring person, someone who wanted to extend his psychiatric interests beyond individual patients to larger social issues. He was at that time not only a clinical professor at the Columbia University College of Physicians and Surgeons, but also an adjunct professor at the Union Theological Seminary and the Columbia Law School—exactly my sort of interdisciplinary soul mate.

Will liked the idea of a center and we immediately shared our knowledge of people and sources of possible money. Will had good contacts in law and medicine, while I had them in philosophy, religion, and the social sciences. Neither of us had ever raised any serious money but, between us, we knew some people who could help. The core of our plan was simple: to organize a nonpartisan, interdisciplinary research and educational organization devoted to ethics and the life sciences.

Apart from finding money and interested participants, our first major organizational question was whether we should aim to become part of a university or remain independent and freestanding. Half of the advice we got favored affiliation ("you'll never make it without a university connection"), while the other half favored independence ("you'll always be trapped by university politics and red tape"). As it happened, I was inclined toward independence, feeling that the field would be stronger, and our center more effective, if we were not seen as an essentially academic enterprise, but worked somewhere back and forth between the general public and the academy. It was noteworthy also that the strongest and most influential research centers—such as the Brookings Institution, the Population Council, the Center for Advanced Study at Princeton, the Urban Institute, and, a bit later, the American Enterprise Institute—were freestanding.

The issue eventually was decided when one of our first benefactors, John D. Rockefeller III, advised us that we would be foolish to become part of a university and to take on all of the problems that doing so would entail. Interestingly, a few other efforts to start bioethics centers at the same time—at Yale and the University of Pennsylvania—did not get off the ground. Never once in 30 years has there been any regret that we remained independent.

## FINDING THE RIGHT PEOPLE

Although finding money was an obvious early worry, much effort went into finding a group of people around the country who were interested in the issues and willing to work with us. How did we find them? We simply asked about, Will and I, each in our own circles. We started with the few people then doing some writing about the issues—Paul Ramsey and James Gustafson among the theologians; Theodosius Dobzhansky, Ernst Mayr, and Rene Dubos among the scientists; Renee C. Fox and Robin Williams among the social scientists; Hans Jonas, Sissela Bok, and K. Danner Clouser among the philosophers; Paul Freund and Harold Green among the lawyers; and Eric Cassell, Fritz Redlich, Robert F. Murray, Jr., and Robert S. Morison among the physicians. Some young people, still in their twenties, were suggested to us as well: Leon R. Kass, then at the National Institutes of Health; Alfred and Blair Sadler, identical twins, one a lawyer and the other a doctor, also at the NIH where they were putting together the Anatomical Gift Act; and Alexander M. Capron, a student of Jay Katz at the Yale Law School.

The initial work of finding people and money took place in 1969 and the early 1970s. Early grants came from the National Endowment for the Humanities, the Rockefeller Foundation, and the Rockefeller Brothers Fund. By early 1970, we had gained our IRS nonprofit status, had a board of directors in place, and were ready to rent our first offices. We moved into an office building in Hastings-on-Hudson in the fall of 1970. Robert M. Veatch, still finishing a Ph.D. at Harvard, was our first staff member, wonderfully productive right from the start. Will Gaylin and I had agreed from the beginning that I would be the full-time CEO of the Center while Will would be a part-time president. It turned out to be a remarkable relationship. Our different skills and interests complemented each other nicely, we rarely had any serious disagreements, and we made a most effective team. Both of us liked our role as entrepreneurs, and we were especially good when working together to gain money.

Our most notable failure was with the Kennedy Foundation, an obvious target for our fund-raising efforts. Though we gave it our best shot, we got nothing from them. Andre Hellegers, who was then beginning the work of founding the

Kennedy Institute at Georgetown, succeeded. I envied Andre's great organizing and fund-raising skills and wished I could do as well. We could have used some of that Kennedy money.

To complement the work of what we assumed would remain a small staff, we created a group of elected "fellows," to be drawn nationwide from the most distinguished workers in the field—though it was a "field" that was not quite a field at that point, well before the term "bioethics" came to be used to describe what we were doing. If that strategy was meant to help us, it was also meant to help them. We thought of the Center's fellowship program as itself important in shaping a field and providing the comparatively few writers and researchers with real colleagues, individuals who were in short supply at most of their home institutions.

I have often been asked whether it was difficult to start the Center. Yes and no. It is "no" in the sense that we did not have to struggle all that hard to find early money, or interested participants; and we had full confidence that, if the venture did not succeed, it would be our fault and not the immaturity of the field or a lack of useful work to do. But it was difficult in one important sense. It was hard at that time to make most educated people believe that ethics is a subject that can be approached with some rigor and produce some useful results. The last wisps of the positivism of the 1940s and 1950s were still present, particularly in medicine, where there are scientific truths, and then there is everything else, mainly emotion or superstition. The fact-value dichotomy was thought permanent and only the fact side of the divide was worth anything. A. J. Ayer (1946), the distinguished Oxford philosopher, pushed that position most effectively in *Language, Truth, and Logic*. Again and again it was obvious how great the impact of that position had been with the generation of physicians, scientists, and foundation functionaries whom we encountered.

The pervasive skepticism about the subject matter was easily matched by doubt about the value of even studying such a soft subject. At most, there was agreement that there were problems of importance and that they could be called ethical in nature. But there was no agreement at all that some adequate measure could be taken of them. That already bad situation was made even worse when ethics came to be seen by some scientists as potentially harmful to scientific progress. Henry Knowles Beecher of the Harvard Medical School (and one of our early fellows) did not endear himself to the medical community in the 1960s when he blew the whistle on wrongful medical research (Beecher 1966). Ethical debate, it was feared, could lead to irrational, fear-driven criticisms of science, further alienating a public that seemed—to the scientists anyway—always on the verge of turning against technology. Doctors were fearful that ethics would engender excessive public criticism, feeding the malpractice virus and diminishing their authority.

It was a constant struggle to deal with those worries. Often enough we got the money we needed, but many of our donors doubted that much would come of our work. The work had to be supported because the problems were real, but that was about the extent of the conviction. Our most notable moral, though not monetary, victory came about in 1974. A grant proposal, submitted by our second professional staff member, Marc Lappé, to look at ethical issues raised by the brand new recombinant-DNA techniques, was rather nastily turned down by the National Institutes of Health. Our concern about the research, we were told, was nothing other than "blue sky philosophizing." By 1975, the same official who said that to us was utterly overwhelmed by the public debate that by then had developed. We never did get a grant, but we did get a rueful apology from him. And sweet it was, (almost) better than the money.

## CHOOSING OUR FOCUS

As time went on, skepticism about bioethics gradually faded—though every few years since then have seen an ethics backlash, the latest in the context of the cloning debate—and the work of the Center progressed. Faced with an intimidating range of issues and a small staff, we felt it would be wise to select a few areas as a focus of our attention. We choose death and dying, genetics, reproductive biology and population issues, and behavior control.

We assumed those areas would remain of importance in the years ahead, and, with one exception, we were right. The exception was "behavior control," by which we meant the use of medical and scientific techniques to control, modify, and manipulate human behavior. In the 1970s, considerable research work was going on with psychosurgery, the pharmaceutical control of mood and behavior, and various behavioristic techniques of managing behavior. But the scientific work of the time did not advance in any significant way and, by the end of the 1970s, there seemed little to study. Only in the early 1990s, with the emergence of Prozac and a widening use of Ritalin for attention deficit disorders, did the topic take on a fresh life and open some new research doors for us. Issues of health policy, not nationally prominent in our early days, began to gain some salience in our work by the end of the 1970s, as debates about universal health care, cost control, and rationing became more pronounced.

I do not want to give the impression that our focus was exclusively on bioethics research in the early years. We advertised our mission as "research and education," and we meant it. One of our first educational projects was to help foster the introduction of ethics into medical school curricula, beginning with such an effort at the College of Physicians and Surgeons at Columbia University in 1971.

That endeavor was a mixed success. We did get some ethics segments introduced into a few courses and managed to sponsor some lectures and discussion groups. But we came a political cropper when one of the medical students we were teaching chose to talk in our class about Columbia's failure to have a dialysis unit and the problems that was causing. The administration of the medical school, embarrassed by such discussion under the rubric of "ethics," quickly saw us as troublemakers (not our intention) and medical ethics as a source of exposes of hospital and physician failure (not our aim at all).

Our trouble was compounded when Will Gaylin (1972) wrote an article for the *New York Times Magazine* on cloning. It was hardly a lurid article, but it managed to enrage the dean of the medical school, who said that Will's article would do harm to biomedical research and the ability of the medical school to raise money. That was the end of us at Columbia, but in 1972 we held a large and highly successful conference on the teaching of ethics in medical schools. By then the teaching of ethics was beginning to spread quite rapidly, and within a few years it was a prominent enough development to make any further work on our part superfluous.

Our more sustained educational efforts came with a series of summer workshops on bioethics in the 1970s; the establishment of a visiting scholar program; and, most importantly, the creation of the *Hastings Center Report* in mid-1971 *(Hastings Center Report* 1971). Weren't there already too many journals in the world, we were asked? Probably so we responded, but we needed an outlet for some of our research and we believed the field was ripe for a journal. It was a good move. The *Report* soon became the leading journal in bioethics, a status greatly facilitated of course by the absence of any other journals at all throughout most of the 1970s. What the *Report* most effectively succeeded in doing was to demonstrate that there could be solid, interesting, and helpful analysis and writing about ethics. That fact, together with the workshops and visiting scholar programs, helped considerably in establishing the credentials of bioethics, thereby allaying many of the worries that initially had been voiced about the enterprise.

As the Center developed during its early years, a number of events were taking place in the field of bioethics to raise the latter's stature and increase its influence. In the summer of 1974, the philosopher Samuel Gorovitz organized a conference at Haverford College that brought together a large number of philosophers drawn to the field. Until that time, the major figures from ethics tended to have a religious and theological background. The entrance of the philosophers radically tilted the field in a secular direction. This shift was not simply because most of the philosophers were not religious, but more tellingly because they had little use for the theologians and their style of ethical discourse, which they labeled vague, fuzzy, and latently sectarian, not up to the rigorous standards of a more public role for bioethics. After the mid-1970s, I had a constant struggle (which never really ended) to get the philosophers among our fellows even to tolerate theologians at our project meetings: "what's the point?" they said.

## THE SECULARIZATION OF BIOETHICS

What might be called the secularization of the field was given an even sharper nudge by the establishment of the National Commission for the Protection of Human Subjects in 1974, in great part because of the interest of Senator Walter Mondale, one of our first fellows (United States Congress 1973). Although the ethical problems of human subjects research provided the main impetus for the Commission, its work gave bioethics considerable visibility and placed a premium on developing the language and way of thinking about bioethics that would carry weight in the public sphere. It was the secular philosophers together with the lawyers in the field who provided those ingredients. The theologians continued to be read for a time, but their influence gradually diminished. The *Belmont Report*, a product of the work of the National Commission (1979), helped to advance the moral theory that became known as principlism, which in turn was further advanced by the work of Tom Beauchamp and James Childress (1979) in their influential book *Principles of Biomedical Ethics*, now in its fourth edition. The establishment of the President's Commission for the Study of Ethical Problems in Medicine and Biomedical and Behavioral Research in 1979, led by Morris Abrams as Chairman and Alexander M. Capron as Executive Director, helped to round out the decade of the 1970s, giving still more prominence to bioethics.

While the Hastings Center had no direct involvement in the work of the two commissions, there is little doubt that they helped our mission. As time went on, it became easier to raise money for the Center, particularly from the large national foundations. The Commonwealth Fund, the Ford Foundation, the Kaiser Family Foundation, and the New York Foundation became active supporters, while the various Rockefeller Foundations continued the support that had been there from the beginning. It might be noted parenthetically that none of those foundations regularly continued to provide bioethics grants after the 1980s, to us or to anyone else. Bioethics came and went as agenda items for them.

Most strikingly, and a source of puzzlement, was the great difficulty of gaining grants from the large health-oriented foundations. The Robert Wood Johnson Foundation, the Kellogg Foundation, the Pew Charitable Trusts, and, later, the Commonwealth Fund of the 1980s seemed utterly disinterested in ethics. Their focus was on empirical studies and demonstration projects in health care, neither of which we did. It was a source of some ironical bemusement on my part that the

Robert Wood Johnson Foundation accorded me the nice honor of asking me to speak to their staff from time to time about my own writings, but I got nowhere when I tried to get a grant from them, although I can report that there has been some improvement since then.

As I tried to understand that situation, it gradually occurred to me that there were two groups of professionals with an almost systematic disinterest in ethics: economists and quantitatively oriented health policy analysts. They were the principal recipients of the grants from the health-oriented foundations, and often enough the staff members of those foundations were trained in those fields. And if it can be said that there is a mainstream health policy establishment, then it is fair to say it is dominated by disciplines that tend to bypass ethics altogether. The great triumph of bioethics was to gain a serious place at the table in clinical medicine. Its great failure has been its inability to even sit for long stretches in the kitchen of the health policy field; only a recent interest in equitable distribution of health care resources, and a few side issues, has slightly opened that door.

I so far have paid most attention to the administrative and financial development of the Center. That focus seems to me not nearly as interesting or important as the Center's intellectual development, and particularly the manner in which that development has influenced and interacted with the like development of the field.

## INTERDISCIPLINARY IDEALS

From the first, the Center was dedicated to interdisciplinarity. Two points were essential to that commitment. One of them was that the issues of the field, whether birth, life, or death, should always be looked at through the prism of every discipline that had something of pertinence to say. A corollary conviction was that no single discipline could claim to have a privileged status in the analysis of ethical issues. That conviction led directly to the second, related point: ethical analysis should take a problem from the ethical level through the policy and legal levels, and each of these levels should interpenetrate the others.

To fulfill that commitment, the Center over the years has always had a diverse staff: philosophers; lawyers; clinicians (though not many and never full time); psychologists and anthropologists; theologians; and political scientists. It has not, however, ever had an economist, or a sociologist, or a demographer, or a bench scientist. My own working principle over the years was that, if possible, every staff member should have at least one colleague from his own field (to have someone to talk shop with) but that no field should ever have more than two representatives, lest their shop talk come to dominate the general discourse. That principle has worked out well, and there has never been any feeling among the staff that one field had a privileged position. It has however become harder in recent years to keep the staff interested in the whole range of bioethics issues, more characteristic of the earlier years. They seemed pushed toward, or maybe attracted by, more specialized focus on one or two sets of problems (genetics or care of the dying, for instance) and defend themselves by saying that the field is more complex now and that no one person can be on top of it all.

If our ideal has been one of interdisciplinarity, my impression is that the field in general has gravitated to a kind of oligopoly of fields. Philosophy, law, and medicine are now the dominant disciplines. Clinical medicine has generated many of the key problems of interest to the field; philosophy has contributed the analytical, secular style of reasoning preferred in the field; and law has been vital since so many of the issues take a legal turn. The Center worked more closely in its early years with historians than it currently does. It is rare now for the *Hastings Center Report* to have a historical article submitted, and few of its recent research groups have sought the aid of historians. That is unfortunate.

The relationship with the social sciences has always been somewhat troubled. On the one hand, many in bioethics feel that there has been a kind of *resentment* toward bioethics among medically oriented social scientists: a feeling perhaps that bioethics has displaced them a bit on medical faculties, or that bioethicists do not take their insights and methods seriously enough, or do not take the trouble to understand the value of social science perspectives for ethics. And it has been true that those in bioethics have not exactly rushed to the social sciences as part of their effort to understand ethical problems and their social setting (in great part because the reigning analytical style of moral philosophy is not much interested in that). Under the influence of philosophy, there has been at least a latent view that, since an "ought" cannot be derived from an "is," social science knowledge cannot in the end be decisive for the making of moral judgments. That may be true, if "decisive" is the key word, but that does not preclude many other instructive insights the social sciences can offer before reaching that point.

Whatever the possible reasons for the tension between bioethics and the social scientists, there are some suggestions that it is abating a bit as bioethicists show more interest in social context and cultural differences. But there may never be a full meeting of minds between those who see their work as developing sound moral judgments about right and wrong, good and bad, and those who see their vocation as providing informed descriptions and explanations of actual practices and mores. Each may need the other but it is not yet fully clear just *how* they need each other.

Although there have, then, been ongoing problems between philosophers and theologians, and bioethicists and social scientists, they are easily matched by what I see as the greatest fissure in the field, at least for me. It is a fissure that circles me back to those other tensions. There have been, I suggest, at least two distinct streams in bioethics from the start, both valid and important but distinctly different from one another. One of them took its point of departure from the abuses and problems originally identified by Beecher, centering on the protection of individuals from abusive biomedical research, and broadening out from there to encompass the rights of patients, informed consent, self-determination in medical treatment and the termination of that treatment, and a wide range of difficult dilemmas concerning the vulnerable and those of diminished competence. I will call this the autonomy movement, emphasizing the need to protect the vulnerable, to empower the competent, and to find a better balance between doctor and patient than that represented by the traditional paternalism of the Hippocratic tradition. Its fullest expression can, I suspect, be found in the moral theory of principlism, in which the principles, when they are parsed, all come back to autonomy, the most powerful and dominating of the principles. This was bioethics as the natural child of American individualism.

## BIOETHICS AND CULTURE

The other stream is somewhat more difficult to characterize, but might best be called cultural. It was interested in the way medical developments and technologies would affect our thinking about human nature and culture; and how that thinking, and the ways of life it could create, should be judged. Where would the technological developments take human life, individually and socially? What kind of society, and with what moral values, might medical advances and technology generate?

What would human cloning do to our ideas about personal identity? What would a capacity of medicine to allow us to predetermine the sex of our children do to those children—and to the idea and values of childbearing and child rearing? What kind of society, and what kind of families, would result from efforts to bypass traditional means of procreation? Or to radically increase average life expectancy? Could one—in the face of an autonomy-driven ethics, and a view of public policy that put the right before the good—generate a rich discussion of the trajectory of biomedical research and innovations, focused on their societal impact and social meaning and not just their implications for individual needs and desires? I have written in other places of the three ways in which medical advances have introduced change (Callahan 1998). They first changed our conception of the role and possibilities of medicine, then our understanding of human health, and then our thinking about the living of a life. A full-bore bioethics would seek to explore all three of these dimensions.

To some extent that has happened, but far less than I had hoped as the Center was getting underway. The other stream, with its endless, legally charged focus on individual choice and welfare, has been dominant. It is prone to be immediately practical in its aims and reductionist in its methods, looking to a right, or a principle, or a rule, to cut through ethical puzzles. In part I suspect that is because the larger questions are less congenial to analytically inclined philosophers, to policy experts, to legislators, and to lawyers. The marginalization of religion in bioethics effectively downgraded one potential source of vigor to explore the larger questions, and the ongoing strain with the social sciences tended to stifle the possibilities that a more effective collaboration could bring about.

Although they have always had a following, the work of such Center fellows as Leon R. Kass, William F. May, Gilbert Meilaender, David Smith, Hans Jonas, and perhaps myself has always been slightly out of the mainstream. It was a source of considerable disappointment to me that my mid-1990s project on "the goals of medicine" captured far less interest in this country than in Europe. I have long been convinced that we cannot effectively come to grips with problems of aging, resource allocation, justice, and the medicalization of many social pathologies without a renewed debate on the goals of medicine. Moreover, it seemed to me only logical that medical education should begin and end with a serious examination of medical goals: what is it we are trying to do? In any case, I have not been able to generate the enthusiasm for that topic I had hoped for. It seems to go against a tide that is more interested in means than in ends.

That point touches on my main objection to principlism. It is not that the principles are necessarily the wrong ones, or that there is no good method for reconciling conflicts among them (the standard objections). Instead, it is that they have served most effectively a kind of blocking function. By providing a relatively easy method to solve many ethical problems, and by being only too well adapted to Anglo-American culture, principlism has in practice (if not necessarily in its theory) short-circuited the opening up of larger, more important issues. Principlism has, for instance, surely led to a robust, dominating moral role for autonomy in bioethics, but it offers no guidance whatever about how to use our freedom or what counts as a good exercise of autonomy. The right to make a choice is regularly confused with the goodness of a choice, two utterly separate matters. Justice is an important principle, but it generally is understood simply as a necessary means to help people achieve equal opportunity in the pursuit of autonomy. Beneficence has never, save with some religiously inclined thinkers, had much moral status. It requires coming to some judgment about what is good for people—exactly the kind of judgment that an autonomy driven culture works hard to avoid (even declaring, in "thin" theories of the good, that it can be dangerous). Nonmaleficence is readily acceptable because it is usually reduced to the avoidance of physical harm to individuals. But what would count as nonmaleficence in our stance toward society, toward cultural traditions, toward settled ways of life? The principle of nonmaleficence has rarely been understood as one that should lead us to ask such questions.

## WHAT HAVE WE WROUGHT?

Perhaps the most astounding part of the early years of the Hastings Center was the rapidity with which it grew and with which the field of bioethics caught on. We had expected to have, at most, a staff of four or five when the Center reached full strength and a budget of less than $500,000 a year. By the end of the 1970s, our staff had reached 15 and our budget was nearing $1 million. That early staff included Arthur Caplan, Ruth Macklin, and Thomas Murray, all of whom, along with Robert Veatch, became leaders of other bioethics centers. Our summer workshops in the 1970s provided a large number of people with their first systematic introduction to bioethics. The *Hastings Center Report* had established itself as the leading journal in the field, as had *IRB: A Review of Human Subjects Research* (still the only journal devoted to that topic). Our assorted research projects led to a large number of books and articles, which we like to think made a serious contribution to the field and to public policy. The field of bioethics blossomed and grew, picked up by the media, adopted by medical and nursing schools, pursued even at the undergraduate level where courses in bioethics proved to be immensely popular with students. The National Institutes of Health, slow in the early years to support bioethics, finally began providing grants (principally through the Human Genome Project) and intensified its efforts at its clinical center. Just about every professional organization in medicine created study groups, or committees, or mechanisms of one kind or another to put bioethics on their agenda.

I could go on and on about what happened to the field, but that's enough. All along the way the Hastings Center has been an active and central actor. So, what have we wrought? I have some mixed feelings about that. We surely accomplished institutionally what we had set out to do: to help put bioethics on the national intellectual and academic map; to provide forums and occasions for debate and discussions; to advance professional and public education; and to publish useful articles and books. Indeed, we far exceeded our own expectations in that respect, not only because of the early success of our own work but also because we were riding the crest of a wave much larger and more intense than we ever anticipated.

But I have some serious misgivings as well, not all of which are easy for me to put my finger on. I will begin with one perhaps small but nonetheless telling phenomenon: a fair number of us who have been in the field for a number of years feel a bit embarrassed to describe ourselves as "ethicists" or "bioethicists," something I discovered when I began asking various colleagues how they felt about those terms. Most of them prefer to use more settled disciplines by which to identify themselves, such as philosopher, or theologian, or physician. It is as if we are not sure whether bioethics as a field is quite as solid or distinguished or important as many other, more established fields; and perhaps we also feel that the media and professional attention gained by bioethics is greater than its actual accomplishments. I can only speculate here, since those who share this wariness about using the more common terms are not always fully able to say why they feel that way.

I also think it fair to say that, despite the pervasiveness of courses in colleges and professional schools, and the no less pervasive outpouring of articles in leading journals, bioethics has not established itself all that well in the higher reaches of the academy. Despite gaining a solid place in most medical schools, it is still something of an outsider, one of those hybrid fields (such as American studies, or urban studies, or ethnic studies) that is seen as second-rate in comparison with more focused, single-discipline fields. In one sense, this is no doubt because interdisciplinary studies have never achieved a high status in universities. But in another sense, it may well be that this particular interdisciplinarity is so broad and unwieldy that it has even more of an uphill struggle.

Yet even as I note this fact, for so I think it is, I am ambivalent: I continue to think interdisciplinary work is of equal importance with classical disciplinary work, and I take it to be a great strength of the field that it has held on to that feature (even if the range of key disciplines has diminished a bit since the 1970s). But it is quite clear that not everyone shares that conviction—not the traditional disciplines, which tend to look down their noses at bioethics; nor the major foundations, only a few of which have ever seen fit to make bioethics a settled and strong program area (the Greenwall Foundation and one or two others being the rare exceptions); nor the most distinguished learned societies and scientific societies, which are not rushing to elect us to their ranks.

Oddly enough perhaps, even as the field fails to establish itself as a first-rank intellectual discipline, bioethics has moved a long way toward becoming a substantial sub-discipline, with many of the same trappings as those that are more established. It now has a plethora of journals, most of which nervously want to explain that, just like the big guys, they are peer review journals. Being such a journal means of course that one can safely list publications in them on one's CV, thus helping the anxious quest for tenure and other prizes. It also means that, like most disciplinary or sub-disciplinary work, there are a large number of citations

to other specialists in the discipline, a kind of herd mentality in pursuing the rec-
ognizably "hot" topics of the moment, and the kind of subdued emotions and flat
prose thought appropriate to serious academic writing.

I find this rather sad on balance, bespeaking too often not the excitement and
pleasure of pursuing subjects of interest and importance, but a deep-seated worry
about pleasing one's colleagues, and taking as few chances as possible lest some
fatal error be made. I wish more young people in bioethics would aspire to write
op-ed articles, to aim for the large monthly magazines like *Harper's* or *The Atlantic
Monthly*, and to publish books aimed at reaching an educated audience, not just
other academics. In saying all of this, I recognize that many of us who were in on
the early days of the Center worked in an era when there were more academic jobs
available, when tenure was easier to obtain, and when there was a greater openness
about writing in an interdisciplinary way for a general audience. So, I can sym-
pathize with my younger colleagues even as I bemoan the results. And the worst
part of it all is that, despite the more academic and disciplinary turn of the field, it
seems not to make a whit of difference in increasing the field's academic stature; if
anything it makes the field more and more of an academic ghetto.

The final misgiving I will mention brings me back to themes touched on above,
the tension with religion and the social sciences, for one thing, and with the pursuit of the larger cultural questions, for another. But this time I want to point to
the strain of ideological thinking that has inserted itself into the field over the
years. Religious and political conservatives regularly complain that the field is
generally liberal, and predictably so, in its ideological leanings. Although I often
bridle at large generalizations of that kind, knowing of too many exceptions, it is
a reasonably accurate charge. Although I think we have done reasonably well with
the *Hastings Center Report* over the years in publishing a balanced set of perspectives, many of our critics do not feel that way.

It is surely fair to say that we have not pursued more conservative voices with
the zeal we might—but I can also say that, in their clannishness and with their
liberal-bashing proclivities, conservatives do not send us much to publish, prefer-
ring I suppose more congenial journals of a like mind. In any event, it is not that
we turn down conservative articles more quickly than liberal articles—we just do
not get the conservative articles to consider at all. I have long been sorry about
that, for we could be inspiring and assisting a richer cultural dialogue and not
becoming just another instance of the culture wars. Since many of the conservative voices are religious rather than secular, the bias of the field against religious
viewpoints further opens up what is an unnecessary and debilitating gap. I do not
know if a better relationship with the social sciences would provide something
of an antidote here, but it would surely help to better adumbrate the depth and
reach of religious values in the shaping of American values. Having said all that,

however, I want to add one point: if there are signs of the larger society's culture wars in bioethics, the field, nevertheless, has remained remarkably friendly and generally irenic. The feuds and fights are subdued, and I know of few serious enmities or the kind of outright hostilities that mark many fields. I consider that a great gift and hope it stays that way.

## References

Ayer, Alfred Jules. 1946. *Language, Truth and Logic*. London: V. Gollancz, Ltd.

Beauchamp, Tom L., and Childress, James F. 1979. *Principles of Biomedical Ethics*. New York: Oxford University Press. (Fourth edition published by Oxford in 1994.)

Beecher, Henry K. 1966. Ethics and Clinical Research. *New England Journal of Medicine* 274: 1354–1360.

Callahan, Daniel. 1970. *Abortion: Law, Choice, and Morality*. New York: Macmillan.

Callahan, Daniel. 1998. *False Hopes*. New York: Simon & Schuster.

Gaylin, Willard. 1972. The Frankenstein Myth Becomes a Reality: We Have the Awful Knowledge to Make Exact Copies of Human Beings. *New York Times Magazine* (5 March, Section 6, Part 1): 12–13, 41, 43–44, 48–49.

*Hastings Center Report*. 1971. *Hastings Center Report* 1 (June).

National Commission for the Protection of Human Subjects of Biomedical and Behavioral Research. 1979. The Belmont Report: Ethical Principles and Guidelines for the Protection of Human Subjects of Research. *Federal Register* 44 (18 April): 23192–23197.

Rawls, John. 1971. *A Theory of Justice*. Cambridge, MA: Belknap Press.

United States Congress. 1973. Senate. Committee on Labor and Public Welfare. Subcommittee on Health. Quality of Health Care—Human Experimentation, Parts 1–4: Hearings before the Subcommittee on Health, 93rd Congress, 1st Session, February-March. Washington, DC: U.S. Government Printing Office.

# 2

# A MEMOIR OF AN
# INTERDISCIPLINARY CAREER

It was the late 1960s, searching about for a professional niche in life, that I became interested in the emerging ethical and policy problems of what was then called "the biological revolution," but could no less have been called the "medical revolution."

Where was biology taking us? In the air were utopian speculations about remaking human nature, allowing us to choose the genetic characteristics of our children, and radically extending human life expectancy. How should we ethically assess those possibilities? At the same time, complaints were rising about medicine's power to keep us alive too long and too miserably, anxieties were emerging about the rising costs of health care, and revelations were surfacing about wrongful exploitations of human beings for research purposes. How should those issues be evaluated?

## CREATION OF THE HASTINGS CENTER

With such questions in mind, in 1969 I helped create a research center devoted to the ethical and policy problems of medicine and biology. It was eventually called the Hastings Center, named after the town in which we started, Hastings-on-Hudson, NY (Callahan 1999). I recruited a neighbor to work with me, Willard

Gaylin, a psychiatrist who had been an English major at Harvard before going into medicine, and the author of interesting books on various social problems having little to do with the technical problems of psychoanalysis, his specialty. So far as I know, he never wrote a single article for professional journals in psychiatry, but managed to make a solid name for himself in the field, and far beyond it. For my part, I had a PhD in philosophy, focused on moral philosophy. We made a fine interdisciplinary pair.

Not only because of our own proclivities, but also because of the breadth of the issues, we quickly agreed that our Center, and the field (still to be created), should be interdisciplinary. I was at that time working with demographers at The Population Council in New York on the ethical problems of trying to lower birth rates in developing countries; that was my introduction to demography and reproductive biology. Gaylin, meanwhile, had simultaneous appointments at the Columbia University College of Physicians and Surgeons, Union Theological Seminary, and the Columbia University School of Law, an uncommon mix.

How did I become interested in interdisciplinary work? I have to go back in my personal history to explain that. As an undergraduate at Yale in the late 1940s I was unsure what field interested me the most. Then Yale created what it called an "interdisciplinary major," allowing students to take a variety of courses but without any single disciplinary focus or any effort to coordinate the courses one took. My combination was literature, history, and psychology. It was not much of a program, and was subsequently improved with seminars and course coordination. But it was quite enough to wet my interdisciplinary appetite.

I finally decided on graduate work in philosophy, though I had only one philosophy course as an undergraduate. I chose the Harvard philosophy department, then in the throes of Oxford-dominated analytic philosophy. Along the way to getting my degree I taught a freshman writing course and also served as a research assistant to a cultural historian. By the time I received my degree I decided I was not enthralled with analytic philosophy and particularly its narrow approach to ethics; nor did I see myself settling down in an academic philosophy department. My work with historians made me acutely aware of the cultural setting of ideas, and how even analytic philosophy was the child of a special Anglo-American outlook on philosophy, narrowly indifferent to other ways of thinking and insensitive to the unexamined culture that had shaped it.

Instead of teaching, I then took a job in New York as a magazine editor, a position I kept for 7 years. I wanted to make some use of my philosophy education, but outside of the university; that desire—combined with my interest in medicine and health care—led to the idea of starting the Hastings Center. The combination of my own checkered academic and journalistic life, and the nature of the field we were shaping—which came to be known as bioethics—made the need for inter-disciplinary work obvious.

Why was interdisciplinarity necessary for bioethics? After all, its focus is on eth-ics, a standard academic discipline in philosophy and religious studies. It seemed to us, however, that the ethical problems emerging from medicine and biology required that they be set in a wide context, not only to understand them well but no less to see the way they played out in the wider world (Callahan 1973).

Our first project was on the changing definition of death, which was then mov-ing from death traditionally defined as the cessation of heart and lung activity to the cessation of whole brain electrical activity. The change was being driven by two forces. One of them was that new technologies were able to keep hearts and lungs going for indefinite periods of time, making it unclear when to stop treatment. The other was that the fast-developing technology of organ transplantation made it necessary to have a more precise definition of death, one that decisively allowed treatment to be stopped, thus making transplantation morally acceptable.

Or did it? Our research project aimed to look at this change to determine how morally valid the move from one definition to another was, and particularly to examine whether the desperate desire for transplantable organs was seductively shaping the debate in a dangerous way. We put together an interdisciplinary team of philosophers and theologians (to include their modes of dealing with ethics); neurologists (to help us understand the concept of brain death); lawyers (to deter-mine how laws and regulations needed to be changed to deal with the new defi-nition); physicians (to understand the implications of the change for the care of dying patients); sociologists and psychologists (to get a sense of how the public would react to the new definition, and whether it would help or hinder the pro-curement of organs); and medical historians (to grasp the history of definitions of death and the force of the symbolic move from the heart to the brain as the locus of death) (Pernick 1999).

It was a fine and interesting exercise, with each of the participants learning from the others. It led to articles in medical, law, and social science journals as well as contributions to public policy in effecting the changed definition. Yet it had already become clear that perhaps our success with that first project was a fluke. Other efforts were not so easy. We were asked to initiate a course in med-ical ethics at a major New York medical school. That sounded interesting and we agreed to do so. Problems quickly surfaced. What kinds of credentials were necessary to teach such a course? Physicians said that obviously they should be the teachers since one could hardly teach such a course without actual medical experience in caring for patients, and that, anyway, to teach ethics was in the end to shape character and that no formal education in ethics was necessary to do that; good role models would do the job. Those with a training in ethics said that ethics was itself a discipline, one that required far more analytical skills than simply serving as a role model.

The compromise solution was to have team teaching, a doctor and a philosopher, sometimes supplemented by a social scientist or nurse. As time went on, however, it gradually became acceptable to have either a physician only, or a philosopher only to teach such courses. It came to be understood that the teacher should have a good disciplinary background in one field but be an educated amateur in the other: a physician teacher should have some education in ethics, and a moral philosopher should understand reasonably well what it was like to practice medicine and understand its culture.

But that was not the end of the problems. Some people held that while the field should be interdisciplinary in the end one field should have a privileged position. Not surprisingly, philosophers believed that their discipline deserved that position and doctors that theirs should. That argument has more or less faded away now, but that is perhaps because the earlier interest on the part of philosophers in the field has cooled considerably. During the 1970s moral philosophy took a more applied form, with the journal *Philosophy and Public Affairs* leading the way. Of late that interest appears to have faded. A larger number of physicians and lawyers are entering the field as the number of philosophers seems to have declined. Bioethics remains a fringe branch of philosophy, widely taught but with no special prestige, and in some departments not taught at all (at Yale, for instance, where I have a "senior scholar" appointment but do not teach).

Another problem was that, in medical schools, there were no departments ready-made for those hired to teach ethics. In what have been called "convenience appointments," various medical departments were willing to give them a home. But when the time came for promotions and tenure decisions, matters often got complicated. If they were housed in, say, the department of surgery, the standards of judgment in surgery would not make sense. Yet if they were philosophers, but not in the philosophy department (much less doing standard philosophy research), that department was not in a position to evaluate them either. Who then were their peers, able to judge their research and teaching (see Holbrook, Chapter 22 this volume)? A common answer was to make use of ethicists at other institutions, doing the same kind of academic work. Moreover, since their work was interdisciplinary, they had to be judged by interdisciplinary, not disciplinary, standards. To ask a philosophy department to use its usual standards of judgment was thought to be unfair. Yet it is probably also fair to say that there are to this day no clear standards about what counts as good interdisciplinary work (see Huutoniemi, Chapter 21 this volume).

While the work of the Hastings Center is carried out by research groups drawn from national talent, that talent has always been interdisciplinary as well: mainly philosophers, lawyers, and social scientists. Staff at Hastings has had to learn how to work with people from other disciplines, understanding their modes of reasoning, their criteria for good work, and the folkways of different disciplines. Three traditions of the staff developed over the years. I told those newly hired that I hoped they would, after a time, learn how to talk in ways that did not reveal their own disciplines; what they said should just sound like ordinary language common sense. That meant, in effect, picking up enough law, philosophy, or social sciences over the years to be able to converse comfortably with experts from those fields—yet without quite sounding like them.

There was also an unwritten rule that no one, under any circumstances, should try to pull disciplinary rank; that is, to claim some special deference in a discussion because of one's discipline. Physicians at our conferences were often the worst offenders, opening their interventions with a sentence that typically began "well, as a physician…," implying that no one but a physician could have the necessary experience and knowledge to say anything of value.

In order to keep interdisciplinarity alive and well at the Center, our hiring practices focused on making certain no one discipline had a disproportionate number. My rule when I was president was that there should be at least one person from every major discipline, but no more than two. Two from a major discipline was the ideal number, so that every staff member would have at least one colleague from the same discipline to talk and work with—but more than two would make it too easy for them to fall into shop talk and not be forced to talk with colleagues in different disciplines. It is a rule that has worked well over the years.

Moreover, as is true with many other free-standing research centers, the fact that we are not part of the university culture—which is heavily organized around disciplinary departments, and with few rewards for serious interdisciplinary work that truly cuts across departments and schools—is a great advantage. My colleagues do not as a rule much care what people in their own disciplines think about them, and they don't feel that they are held hostage by disciplinary peer review. Of course there is a price to be paid for that independence: their work may not be highly thought of by those in their disciplines, in great part because they feel no compunction about working outside of the traditional boundary lines. At the same time it can be said that, though not conforming to disciplinary traditions or worrying much about getting published in peer-reviewed journals, many staff members over the years have been lured away from us to take university jobs.

I have been drawn to interdisciplinary work over the years for some personal and some professional reasons. I like interdisciplinary work because I enjoy reading the literature of different fields, learning things I don't know, and taking on large topics that spill over disciplinary boundaries. Most disciplinary work I think of as painting carefully crafted miniatures: a very careful working through of a small and manageable problem. But I prefer to paint murals and panoramas. And the kinds of panoramas I most enjoy professionally are those that can't be fully assessed without crossing many disciplinary boundaries. The last point can be illustrated by showing how I have approached three major problems in health care in recent years: the clash between government-oriented and market-oriented ideologies in health care reform (Callahan and Wasunna 2006); the control of technology costs in health care (Callahan 2009); and the relationship between birthrates and health care for the elderly (Callahan, manuscript).

## MEDICINE AND THE MARKET IN HEALTH CARE

A key issue in the American debate on health care reform—driven in great part by some 47 million uninsured—is that of the comparative roles that government or the private market should play. If there is to be universal care, should it be put in the hands of the government, which most liberals would like, or should it be managed by private insurers, as most conservatives would prefer? The European health care systems cover all citizens and are either financed directly by government (tax-based systems) or by mandated contributions from employers and employees (social health insurance). Both systems are heavily regulated by government. The American system, *sui generis* among developed countries, is a 50% mix of government financed and managed care and employer-provided private care.

When I first became interested in that issue, I turned to the work of health care economists, who have done research on the performance of both government and private care (Rice 2002). What I wanted to know was the comparative empirical evidence on the market versus government in light of health outcomes, access, quality, and costs. By that standard, European health care systems are easy winners. But as I was reading the economists, I was also following the debate in the pages of *The Wall Street Journal* and other conservative publications and the simultaneous push by President George W. Bush for more private market-driven care. Their test of a good health care system is an ideological one, based on a profound distrust of government and a full embrace of the market. They are far less worried about access and far more worried about consumer choice and private competitive insurers and providers.

The economist heroes of conservatives are Friedrich von Hayek and Milton Friedman, who believed that democracy requires a strong private market, and that a strong private market requires democracy. To understand that ideology requires a grasp of the history of market thinking, going back to Adam Smith.

To understand the specific force of market thinking in the United States I read political scientists, ever returning to Thomas Jefferson who said that "the best government is the least government." To understand the historical resistance of American physicians to a government-run system, it was necessary to understand their objection to any outside force that would interfere with the practice of medicine as they saw fit or threaten their incomes (Starr 1982). To understand the problem of inequity in health care I turned to philosophers, who have given problems of justice a high place. And to understand why health reform has been so difficult to achieve in the United States—with sporadic efforts going back over 60 years—I studied public opinion surveys. They show that a majority of Americans have for years said they favor universal care (75%–80%), but that the surveys also showed profound ideological differences on how it might acceptably be achieved.

Now it may seem self-evident to the reader that if one wants to understand the government-market conflict about health care one should be doing some reading in all those fields. Remarkably enough (and maybe a bit depressingly so) hardly anyone in each of those disciplines cites or makes use of the knowledge or insights from the others. There were exceptions, but those who write on the problem tended to stay within their own disciplines. Health economists do not as a rule cite historians or political scientists and the latter did not cite them. Astonishingly, I was berated by a health care economist for even taking on the topic of medicine and the market, which she believes belongs entirely to her field, and which I as a philosopher have no competence to discuss.

## MEDICAL TECHNOLOGY AND HEALTH CARE COSTS

The United States now spends $2.2 trillion a year on health care. Fueled by a projected 7% cost increase per year for the foreseeable future, the national care costs in a decade will be $4 trillion, some 20% of the gross domestic product. The Medicare program for the elderly, now costing $421 billion a year, will be bankrupt in a decade without radical reform. The rising costs are a major reason for the steady rise of the uninsured, now 47 million, for a decline in employer-provided health care, and for rising out-of-pocket expenses even for those with good health insurance.

While costs rise because of overall inflation pressure and a variety of other causes, the main driver of costs is medical technology, taken to account for 50% of the annual increase (Congressional Budget Office 2008). New technologies and the intensified use of old ones—primarily drugs and medical devices—are the leading accelerants. While many efforts at controlling costs in general and of technology costs in particular have been pursued for over 30 years, none of these efforts have made much difference.

At the heart of the technology problem, I believe, is American culture, one that is uncommonly dedicated to medical progress and technological innovation. American patients seem enamored with progress in general and technology in particular, doctors are trained to use it, and industry makes billions of dollars a year selling it. There are dozens of incentives to use technology in our health care systems, and few disincentives. How is this phenomenon to be understood and dealt with?

While the discipline of health care economics has provided much of the data on rising health care costs as well as offered a solid analysis of its proximate causes, that is simply not enough to get the full picture. Why has Congress forbidden the Medicare program to take cost into account in determining the benefits it will provide for the elderly? That is a question for political scientists and legal scholars. Why is it that compared with other countries, Americans have a much higher respect for medical technology and greater expectations for its benefits? That is a question for medical and cultural historians. The control of costs will of necessity require rationing, not giving patients all they will want and may need. That is a question for philosophers since it must deal with matters of justice, and for legal scholars who will have to cope with the almost certain recourse to the courts by patients denied care. No one of those disciplines can by itself offer a road map to control costs, and at least one reason for a failure to make much progress is the lack of an integrated plan that blends economics, political science, medicine, cultural studies, policy analysis, and ethics.


## BIRTHRATES AND ELDER CARE

Every developed country faces serious problems with a rising number and proportion of the elderly. Health care costs for the elderly under Medicare are shortly projected to rise sharply as the baby boom generation begins to retire, and not too long into the future the Social Security program will come under pressure as well. Yet American problems with an aging society are mild compared with those projected in most other developed countries, where the ratio between the young (whose taxes pay for the old), and the old themselves (who need the financial and social support of the young) is changing to the disadvantage of both the young and the old (United Nations 2004).

At first glance, it might seem that it is medical progress that has greatly lengthened average life expectancy and thus the number of the aged that lies at the root of the cost problem. That is true to some extent (average life expectancy beyond

65 has increased by about 6–7 years since 1970), but a more important influence has been a decline in birthrates. The American baby boom generation (those born between 1947 and 1964) was a very large one, with three or four children for most women. But those baby boomers, now on the verge of retirement, did not themselves have comparably large families, and have been averaging slightly fewer than two children per woman. What had been a ratio of about four younger working people for every retired person is now declining to a ratio of 2.5.

In short, there is a declining base of young taxpayers to support a rising base of elderly retirees. And the situation is far worse in countries like Spain, Italy, Japan, and Poland, where every woman now bears only 1.3–1.4 children. As if the social and medical and economic problems generated by the increased proportion of the elderly is not enough to generate some anxiety, there is considerable agreement among economists that a steady stream of young people is necessary for economic vitality and stability. Many European countries are threatened with declining populations, which will create some unprecedented economic problems (Grant 2004).

To get a good sense of those trends, and to devise public policies to manage them, requires research in a variety of disciplines. I have turned to demographers to get a grasp of the history of procreation and birth rates as well as explanations of various historical trends. Economists have taught me a great deal about the place of young workers in an economy. I make use of historical and sociological knowledge to understand the changing place of family and childbearing in modern societies. Feminists have a good deal to say about governmental calls to increase birth rates and that literature must be consulted. Gerontologists provide important information and studies of the changing place of the elderly in society, as do geriatricians on the medical situation of the elderly. And of course there is a considerable literature—novels, plays, poems—that touch on those topics. To take on the combined topics of bearing children and getting old is to enter a complex, rich, and challenging arena, with hardly any limit to the range of disciplines that can help make sense of it all.


## PASSING IT ON


Looking back on many years of interdisciplinary work, this approach still has an insecure standing in universities and American intellectual life. Interdisciplinary fields and programs in universities are marginal in clout and prestige in comparison with traditional disciplines. I have in mind urban studies, black studies, feminist programs, American studies, and my own field, bioethics. Bioethics now has a place in every medical school, but it hardly has the academic standing of the department of surgery or internal medicine, and it never will. Universities and professional schools are still organized along traditional disciplinary lines, and young faculty members are asking for trouble if they do not publish standard disciplinary articles and research in the mainline disciplinary journals. In what I have come to think of as the tyranny of peer review, CVs frequently now focus on peer-reviewed articles and books, consigning everything else (including op-ed articles in the *New York Times*) to the second-string miscellaneous category, as if it is a kind of waste basket in comparison with the real stuff. It is, however, far harder to get a short article published in the op-ed section of the *New York Times* than a long article in a peer-reviewed journal.

In the early days of the Hastings Center we recruited a number of distinguished scientists—Rene Dubos, Ernst Mayr, Theodosius Dobzhansky, for example—to work with us. For our purposes, they had in common one trait: they had all been educated in Europe, going through the gymnasium system. This meant they had a fine education in the humanities. They were well read, enjoyed mixing it up with philosophers and historians, and were quick to see the important social problems and inclinations of their own research. They had no problem in talking about ethical problems that could well impede scientific research; they were often the first to raise them. They did not treat those from the humanities with skepticism about various scientific developments as enemies of science and research. They thought that is what we are supposed to do.

By the 1990s those distinguished scientists were either dead or retired. The next generation of scientists has been narrower. Their education in the humanities is often scant. Even though it is not necessarily true, applicants to medical schools or PhD programs in biology believe that anything but a straight scientific background in science is a hazard to one's chances of acceptance. Meanwhile, medical and biological research had become more professionally competitive, more expensive, and more grant-driven. A track record of getting grants was not quite as important as publishing in (of course) peer-reviewed journals, but it became a required section on a scientist's CV. Getting grants proves one is a winner, a sign of the right stuff, and a good way to win points in medical schools and science departments always looking for money.

A parallel development began appearing in young applicants for jobs at the Hastings Center. They mainly come out of universities, drawn to us because of a strong reputation in the field. In principle they like our interdisciplinarity, but are nervous about it as well. They have been trained to do rigorous disciplinary work, not to adventurously explore other disciplines. They cannot understand how those of us who were in bioethics in its early years could blithely move from genetics to end-of-life care to health policy to reproductive biology. Why not, I respond: you know how to read, don't you? That casual response rarely persuades them, and the example of those of us who have done just that is often brushed aside. It was easier in the beginning, they respond, but each one of the issues the Center works on is now a large research area with a huge literature; it is unrealistic to expect them to do what we did.

Nonetheless, I continue to chip away at them, noting that there are some old and cross-cutting problems that can be found in the subareas of bioethics. The classical tension between, say, individual good and common good, or medical progress and unforeseen social pitfalls, can be found in almost every discrete topic of bioethics. Over the years, in fact, two distinct streams have emerged in bioethics, going back to its very beginnings, and they have different implications for the field.

One of them, the earliest, came from worries and speculations on the part of leading scientists in the 1960s about where the new biology and medicine were taking us. Would they lead us to think differently about human nature? Would they bring changes in our common life that would lead us to live radically differ-ent kinds of lives than our parents and grandparents? How much power should be granted to science to remake our lives? The other stream focused on some more immediate medical, policy, and legal issues. How can we give patients more autonomy in determining their care at the end of life? Is it possible to establish a better balance of power between doctors and patients? Can we do a better job of protecting research subjects from harm?

Over the years, practical moral problems of that latter kind came to domi-nate the field. The larger initial questions came to be overshadowed. Foundations and the media, among others, were far less interested in the future of humanity under the impact of science than they were of ethics at the bedside, laws on care at the end of life, and specific policy recommendations on stem cell research. The larger speculative questions do not fare well in competition with the more immediate issues, nor do they admit of the land of specificity that can be achiev-ing in devising, say, guidelines for genetic counseling. Interdisciplinary work can and does take place at both levels, but the larger questions are more likely to attract the attention of theologians, a few philosophers, and some stray social scientists. The more policy oriented ones draw on the wider range of disciplines I have noted earlier.

The future of interdisciplinarity in bioethics is not clear. It was easier to pur-sue it in the 1970s than at present, mainly because at the beginning there was no formal field, just a group of people from the biological and medical sciences, the social sciences, philosophy, law, and theology who were interested in the emerg-ing issues, and who saw the value of working together. As time went on and bio-ethics flourished it took on the traits of a subdiscipline and one with increasingly many sub-subdisciplines. At the same time, so it seemed to me, the traditional disciplines became stronger, with pressure on students to stick with the straight and the narrow.

Interdisciplinary work is often lauded as a fine thing, but the underlying message in most universities is to be careful: don't get carried away and don't stray far from established rigor of established disciplines. And if you go into bioethics, pick one area and work at it diligently. Don't flit around from topic to topic. For me, I have to confess the fun and adventure of the field comes in flitting about. I have published only one article in my own field of philosophy, but am far more proud of the fact that I have been published in medical and health policy journals, law reviews, social science journals, science journals, and have had op-ed pieces in every major American newspaper. I have had a good time.

## References

Callahan, D. (1973). Bioethics as a discipline. *Hastings Center Studies* 1(1), 66–73.

Callahan, D. (1999). The Hastings Center and the early years of bioethics. *Kennedy Institute of Ethics Journal 9(l)*, 53–70.

Callahan, D. (2009). *Taming the beloved beast: how medical technology costs are destroying our health care system*. Princeton, NJ: Princeton University Press.

Callahan, D. (manuscript). *Two few babies? The clash of economics, culture, and religion*.

Callahan, D. and Wasunna, A. (2006). *Medicine and the market: equity v. choice*. Baltimore, MD: Johns Hopkins University Press.

Congressional Budget Office (2008). *Technological change and the growth of health care*. Washington, DC: Congressional Budget Office.

Grant, J. et al. (2004). *Low fertility and population aging: causes, consequences, and policy options*. Santa Monica: Rand Corporation.

Pernick, M. (1999). Brain death in a cultural context: the reconstruction of death, 1967–1981. In: S. Youngner, R. Arnold, and R. Schapiro (eds) *The definition of death: contemporary controversies*, pp. 3–33. Baltimore, MD: Johns Hopkins University Press.

Rice, T. (2002). *The economics of health care reconsidered*, 2nd edn. Chicago: Health Administration Press.

Starr, P. (1982). *The social transformation of American medicine*. New York: Basic Books.

United Nations (2004). *Policy responses to population decline and aging*. Population bulletin of the United Nations, special issues 44/45 2002. New York: United Nations.

# 3

---

## MINIMALIST ETHICS

The attraction of morality in affluent times is that not much of it seems needed. More choices are available and thus fewer harsh dilemmas arise. If they do arise, money can be used to buy out of or evade the consequences of choice. The "wages of sin" are offset by the cheapness of therapy, drugs, liquor, economy flights, and a career change. If all else fails, public confessions can profitably be produced as a mini-series. Vice is rewarded because everything is rewarded, even virtue.

Matters are otherwise in hard times. Options are fewer, choices nastier. Where forgiveness and therapeutic labels could once be afforded, blaming and denunciation become more congenial. If life is going poorly, someone obviously must be at fault—if not the government, then my neighbor, wife, or child. The warm, expansive self, indulgent of the foibles of others, gives way to the harsh, competitive self; enemies abound, foreign and domestic. It is not so much that the "least well off" cease to count (though they do), but that most people imagine that they are now in that category. Nastiness becomes the standard of civility; exposé the goal of journalism; a lawsuit the way friends, families, and colleagues reconcile their differences.

Meanwhile, in hard times, every would-be Jeremiah has plentiful material with which to work, and the moral panaceas may be just the opposite of the economic ones. Ethical conservatives want a fatter moral budget: more prayer in more schools, more bombs in more missiles, and more virtue in more hearts to keep more families together. Liberals want a leaner moral budget: less personal moral judgment, less social coercion, and less dominance by the military-industrial-multinational-pharmaceutical-technological expert-Political Action Committee-complex.

What, then, is the problem to be diagnosed? Here is the question I want to ask, and attempt to address: as we move into what will most likely be chronically hard economic times, how can our society muster the moral resources necessary to endure as a valid human culture? Three assumptions underlie that question. The first is that economic strength and military power have no necessary ethical connection with the internal human and moral viability of a culture; they can only help assure its mere existence. The second is that the era of sustained economic growth is over, and with it the perennially optimistic psychology of affluence. The prospects are at best for a steady-state economy, one where the next generation can only hope that it will do as well as the previous generation; only that, no more, and probably less.

My third assumption is that the kind of morality that was able to flourish during affluent times will, if carried over unchanged into hard times, lead to moral chaos and maybe worse. That morality has stressed the transcendence of the individual over the community, the need to tolerate all moral viewpoints, the autonomy of the self as the highest human good, and the voluntary, informed consent contract as the model of human relationships. To be sure, in its "great society" phase, it was a morality sensitive to poverty and economic oppression, just as it more recently supported a quest for universal human rights. But its central agenda was always that of individual liberty, that of the self seeking liberation from both economic and cultural restraints, free to find its own truth and its own way. What is that "truth" and what is the "way"? If you felt you had to ask yourself that question, you probably missed the whole point, failing to use your freedom creatively. If you went so far as to press that question with insistence upon others, you could be certain of some suspicion among those for whom the essential value of autonomy is its resistance to any universal content. Free choice is its own reward, and the philosophical road to hell, supposedly, is paved with teleological ends, ultimate purposes, and essentialist meanings.

Now all of that autonomy is doubtless fine, and lofty, and lovely. But to live that kind of life you need to have money at hand, good health, and a clinic full of psychological counselors at the ready. It is a good-time philosophy for comfortable people living in the most powerful, rich nation on earth. Will it work in hard times? Some doubt is in order.

Hard times require self-sacrifice and altruism—but there is nothing in an ethic of moral autonomy to sustain or nourish those values. Hard times necessitate a sense of community and the common good—but the putative virtues of autonomy are primarily directed toward the cultivation of independent selfhood. Hard times demand restraint in the blaming of others for misfortune—but moral autonomy as an ideal makes more people blameworthy for the harms they supposedly do others. Hard times need a broad sense of duty toward others, especially those out of sight—but an ethic of autonomy stresses responsibility only for one's freely chosen, consenting-adult relationships.

Whether suffering brings out the best or the worst in people is an old question, and the historical evidence is mixed. Yet a people's capacity to endure suffering without turning on each other is closely linked to the way they have envisioned, and earlier embodied, their relationship to each other. When one's perceived and culturally supported primary duty is to others rather than to self, to transcendent rather than private values, to future needs rather than to present attachments, then there can be a solid moral foundation to survive pain, turmoil, and evil. Naturally, that set of values can, and often does, have its dark side. Many nations and cultures serve as unhappy examples of communities that stifled and killed individuals. Tight families and kinfolk systems can run roughshod over liberty, and totalitarian states are all too ready to capitalize upon the willingness of their citizens to give their lives for some higher cause.

What we have not had, until recently, are cultures that have systematically tried to foreswear communal goals; that have tried to replace ultimate ends with procedural safeguards; that have resolutely worked to banish the most profound questions of human meaning to the depths of hidden, private lives only; and that have strived to sanctify the morally autonomous agent as the cultural ideal. Can that kind of a culture survive hard times? Or better, if it is to survive—mere size and residual power may assure that much—can it do so without the wanton violence, moral indifference, and callous self-interest that are the growing pathologies of life in the United States? It would be foolish to give a flat answer to that question. Our cultural experiment is not over. Only now it is faced with a shift in those material circumstances that, as much or more than articulated values, made the culture possible in the first place. The changes will pose a severe test.

## DEFINING THE MINIMALIST ETHIC

One set of moral values that emerged during our recent decades of affluence is peculiarly ill-suited, and even dangerous, for the hard times ahead. For lack of a more graceful term, I will call those values a "minimalistic ethic." I have already hinted at some of the features of that ethic, but will now try to be more specific. That ethic can be stated in a simple proposition: *One may morally act in any way one chooses so far as one does not do harm to others.* The accent and some of the substance of John Stuart Mill's "On Liberty" are familiar enough in that proposition. But something has gone awry in the way Mill's thinking has been appropriated by our culture. What he understood to be a principle that ought to govern only the relationship between the individual and the state has been wrongly construed to encompass the moral life itself.

I call this a "minimalistic ethic" because, put crudely, it seems to be saying that the sole test of the morality of an action, or of a whole way of life, is whether it avoids harm to others. If that minimal standard can be met, then there is no further basis for judging personal or communal moral goods and goals, for praising or blaming others, or for educating others about higher moral obligations to self or community. In the language of our day: the only judgment we are permitted on the way others make use of their moral autonomy is to assess whether they are doing harm to others. If we can discern no such harm, then we must suspend any further moral judgment. Should we fail to suspend that judgment, we are then guilty of a positive violation of their right to privacy and self-determination.

The pervasiveness of this ethic has had a number of general consequences. First, a minimalist ethic has tended to confuse useful principles for government regulation and civil liberties with the broader requirements of the moral life, both individual and communal. Second, it has misled many in our society into thinking that a sharp distinction can be drawn between the public and the private sphere, and that different standards of morality apply to each.

Third, it has given us a thin and shriveled notion of personal and public morality. We are obliged under the most generous reading of a minimalist ethic only to honor our voluntarily undertaken family obligations, to keep our promises, and to respect contracts freely entered into with other freely consenting adults. Beyond those minimal standards, we are free to do as we like, guided by nothing other than our private standards of good and evil. Altruism, beneficence, and self-sacrifice beyond that tight circle are in no sense moral obligations and, in any case, cannot be universally required. My neighbor can and will remain a moral stranger unless and until, as an exercise of my autonomy, I choose to enter into a contract with him; and I am bound to him by no more than the letter of that contract. While I ought to treat my neighbor with justice, that is because I may otherwise do harm to him, or owe it to him as a way of discharging the debt of former injustices, or because it seems a rational idea to develop a social contract with others as a way of enhancing my own possibilities for greater liberty and the gaining of some primary goods.

Fourth, a minimalist ethic has deprived us of meaningful language to talk about our life together outside our contractual relationships. The only language that does seem common is that of "the public interest," a concept which for most translates into the aggregate total of individual desires and demands. The language of "rights" is common enough (though not of putatively archaic "natural" or "God-given" rights). But it is to be understood that the political and moral purpose of both negative and positive rights is to protect and advance individual autonomy. It is not the kind of language that can comfortably be used any longer to talk about communal life, shared values, and the common good.

Fifth, a minimalist ethic has made the ancient enterprise of trying to determine the inherent or intrinsic good of human beings a suspect, probably subversive activity. It assumes that no one can answer such lofty and vague questions, that attempts to try probably pose a threat to liberty, and that, in any event, any purported answers should be left resolutely private.

Sixth, unless I can demonstrate that the behavior of others poses some direct public harm, I am not allowed to question that behavior, much less to pass a public negative judgment on it. The culture of a minimalist ethic is one of rigid and rigorous toleration. Who am I to judge what is good for others? One is—maybe—entitled to personal moral opinions about the self-regarding conduct of others. But a public expression of those opinions would contribute to an atmosphere of moral suppression in the civil order, and of an anti-autonomous moral repression in the private psychological order. One question is taken to be the definitive response to anyone who should be so uncivil as to talk about ethics for its own sake: "But whose ethics?"

In some quarters, a minimalist ethic has gone a step further, to a de-listing of many behavioral choices as moral problems at all. Thus abortion becomes a "religious" rather than a moral issue, and it is well known that all religious issues are private, a-rational, and idiosyncratic; questions of sex, and most recently homosexuality, become matters of "alternative life styles" or "sexual preference"; and the use of pleasure-enhancing drugs becomes an amusing choice between two valued-soaked (subjective) norms, "psychotropic hedonism" or "pharmacological Calvinism."[1]

Seventh, under the terms of a "minimalist ethic" only a few moral problems are worth bothering with at all. The issue of liberty versus justice is one, and that of autonomy versus paternalism is another. The former is important because distributive justice is required to finally enthrone a community of fully autonomous individuals. The latter is vital because it is well recognized that paternalism, even the beneficently motivated and kindly sort, poses the most direct threat to individual liberty. A lack of informed consent, decisions taken by experts, and a failure to observe due process will be high on the list of evils of a minimalist ethic. Anything less than a full egalitarianism—equal decisions made by equally autonomous moral agents—is seen as an eschatological failure.

I have drawn here an exaggerated picture of a minimalist ethic. It fits the views of no one person precisely and, to be sure, cannot be taken to represent any single, coherent, well-developed ethical theory. Not all those who favor a perfect egalitarianism would equally favor (or favor at all) a moral de-listing of matters of sex and drugs. There is no necessary incompatibility between favoring a civil libertarian political ethic and affirming the value of close community ties, of seeking transcendent values and of recognizing duties over and above those of self-realization. Permutations of and exceptions to this general portrait are easy enough to find. Nonetheless, I believe it sufficiently accurate as a composite portrait of a mainstream set of values in American culture to take seriously—and to reject. A society heavily composed of those who aspire to, or unwittingly accept, a minimalistic ethic cannot be a valid human community. In times of stress, it could turn into a very nasty community.

## REREADING MILL

I suggested above that a minimalistic ethic sounds very much like a close relative of John Stuart Mill's position in "On Liberty" (1859), but also that it presses that position beyond the limits he intended. Is that true? I think so, but it is instructive to look at the way Mill tried to find a good fit between principles of public morality, narrow and limited, and the demands of a broader private and communal morality. It is not easy to find that fit, and Mill's troubles in doing so foreshadow many of our own in trying to do likewise. While Mill is by no means responsible for what has transpired in Anglo-American culture since the nineteenth century, his thinking has remained powerful in civil libertarian thought, either as a foundation or as an important point of departure for revised theories.

Recall Mill's famous principle and point of departure in "On Liberty":

> . . . the sole end for which mankind are warranted, individual or collectively, in interfering with the liberty of action of any of their number, is self-protection. That the only purpose for which power can be rightfully exercised over any member of a civilized community, against his will, is to prevent harm to others.[2]

Mill goes on to reiterate and embellish that principle in a variety of ways, stressing not only that society ought to be solely concerned with individual conduct that "concerns others," but also that "over himself, over his own body and mind, the individual is sovereign."[3]

Nor is it sufficient that the individual be protected "against the tyranny of the magistrate."

Protection is also needed, "against the tyranny of the prevailing opinion and feeling; against the tendency of society to impose, by other means than civil penalties, its own ideas and practices or rules of conduct on those who dissent from them. ... There is a limit to the legitimate interference of collective opinion with individual independence: and to find that limit, and maintain it against encroachment, is as indispensable to a good condition of human affairs, as protection against human despotism."[4]

With an even more contemporary flavor, Mill wrote that the principle requires liberty of tastes and pursuits; of framing the plan of our life to suit our own character; of doing as we like, subject to such consequences as may follow: without impediment from our fellow creatures, as long as what we do does not harm them, even though they should think our conduct foolish, perverse, or wrong.[5]

Nevertheless, despite the firmness of those statements, Mill apparently had no desire to reduce all of morality to his "simple principle," as if the moral universe can solely be encompassed by the relationship between the individual and the state. As long as we do not compel anyone in those matters that concern himself only, there can be "good reasons for remonstrating with him, or persuading him, or entreating him ... "[6] So, also, Mill states that

> It would be a great misunderstanding of this doctrine to suppose that it is one of selfish indifference, which pretends that human beings have no business with each other's conduct in life, and that they should not concern themselves about the well-doing or well-being of one another, unless their own interest is involved.... Human beings owe to each other help to distinguish the better from the worse, and encouragement to choose the former and avoid the latter.[7]

Mill's intention, then, is not to promote a society of amoral atoms, each existing in undisturbed isolation from the moral community of others. There are standards of right and wrong, good and bad, in our self-regarding conduct and in our relationship with our fellow creatures—"cruelty of disposition," "malice," "envy," "pride," "egotism," "rashness," and "obstinacy" are all vices for Mill. Yet he is walking a delicate line. He wants to exclude legal pressures in that which concerns ourselves only, and exclude as well "the moral coercion of public opinion." Yet, he also agrees that so long as the individual is the final judge, "considerations to aid his judgment, exhortations to strengthen his will, may be offered to him, even obtruded on him, by others. ... "[8]

I find it difficult to see as sharp a distinction as Mill does between exhorting and obtruding upon others, and allowing them to be free of "the moral coercion of public opinion." It is just that exhortation by others that may and probably will represent public opinion. So what if I am allowed in the end to be my own moral judge? If others insist upon their right to harangue, bother, and even condemn me with their moral sentiments, my fife is considerably less well off—on one reading of Mill—than if they would just let me alone.[9] Moreover, this is exactly what many say in our day: "It is not enough that you grant me the legal and civil liberty to act as I see fit. You must also grant me that private respect and equality that will lead you to stop judging altogether my moral actions."[10]

Much of what Mill says in "On Liberty" would seem to reject that latter extension of his "simple principle." For him, the problem of his day was not too much individuality, but too little. One can only read with a kind of wondrous bemusement a passage like the following:

> ...the danger which threatens human nature is not the excess, but the deficiency, of personal impulses and preferences. ...In our times, from the highest class of society down to the lowest, everyone lives as under the eye of a hostile and dreadful censorship. ...It does not occur to them to have any inclination, except for what is customary.[11]

If one worked at it, I suppose, one could still find many in our society who have no inclination except for what is customary. There are allegedly one or two people like that on my street and many more, I have been assured, living in the Sun Belt, Palm Springs, and Scarsdale. But how do we determine what counts as "customary" any longer in a society that allows any and all moral flowers to bloom?

Mill is not unaware of the possibility that the kind of liberty he seeks can lead to some undesirable outcomes:

> I fully admit that the mischief which a person does to himself may seriously affect, both through their sympathies and their interests, those nearly connected with him and, in a minor degree, society at large[12]. ...But with regard to the merely contingent, as it may be called, constructive injury which a person causes to society, by conduct which neither violates any specific duty to the public, nor occasions hurt to any assignable individual except himself: the inconvenience is one which society can afford to bear, for the sake of the greater good of human freedom.[13]

In another place, he writes that "mankind are greater gainers by suffering each other to live as seem good to themselves, than by compelling each to live as seems good to the rest."[14]

That may be too confident and optimistic a judgment. What societies did Mill have in mind when he came to that conclusion? Apparently not his own or any other extant society. In the passage quoted above, for instance, those societies were characterized as repressive and conformist. He must have been extrapolating from some parts, or circles, of his own social world to have reached such a universal judgment. Yet only in our day have we actually begun to see an approximation, on a mass scale, of the kind of society he had in mind. Lacking other historical examples, it is those we must judge. Whatever its other failings, Mill lived in a time and a culture that could take many if not most Western moral values for granted. He did not have to specify or defend the standards by which his countrymen should judge the self-regarding behavior of others, or the moral principles to be inculcated in children, or the norms on which the moral exhortation he countenanced was based.

## PUBLIC AND PRIVATE MORALITY

Increasingly, no such background—tacitly held and almost superfluous to state—can be assumed. Precisely because that is so, and because a minimalist ethic has been one outcome of the train of thought that Mill helped set in motion, we are forced to now re-examine the relationship between public and private morality. Can they, in the first place, sharply be distinguished, as Mill thought possible?

The evidence provided by the emergence of a minimalist ethic is hardly encouraging. Not only would it have us obsessively make such a distinction; it would have us go a step further and eschew moral judgment on the private lives of others as well. In response, I want to argue three points. First, the distinction between the private and the public is a cultural artifact only, varying with time and place. Second, only a thoroughly dulled (or self-interested) imagination could even pretend to think that there can be private acts with no public consequences. Third, the effort to sharply distinguish the two spheres can do harm to our general moral life.

What kind of human nature, and what kind of society, would be necessary to viably and sensibly separate the private and the public sphere? As for human nature, the individual would have to exist in total isolation from all others, dependent upon them for nothing at all, neither food, shelter, culture, nor language. If a universe existed that made possible that kind of individual, one might then speak of a wholly private, inward world. But the concept of a "public" world would then make no sense. There would be none of those interconnections and interdependencies, past, present, and future human relationships, that characterize what is ordinarily meant by "public." In such a universe, it would also be hard to make much sense of "human nature." It would lack those traits, language, and culture in particular, reasonably thought necessary to distinguish the "human" from other forms of nature.

If we leave that never-never universe, and ask what kind of society would have to be imagined to support a sharply separable private and public space, our task might seem a bit easier. Do we not, after all, have our secret thoughts, and do things that others never hear about or see? Of course, but what does that prove? As Mill himself acknowledges, actions have their cause in internal dispositions,[15] precisely within the hidden self. While our behavior can belie our secret thoughts and feelings some of the time, it is difficult to imagine a constant discrepancy between the inner and the outer self. One way of coming to know our inner self, it often turns out, is by observing our outer self, that self which acts and responds in the company of others; it is normally impossible to say just where the one begins and the other ends. Aristotle's observation that virtue is a habit was not unperceptive, nor is it any the less consonant with general experience to suggest that our habits of private thought, our hidden feelings and dispositions toward others, have a direct bearing on observable conduct, on our habits.

One need not turn to the complicated relationship between an inner and an outer self to wholly make the point. Our more recent historical experience indicates that the distinction between the public and the private is at the least a cultural artifact and quite possibly a matter of the sheerest ideology. I earlier pointed to a "de-listing" phenomenon in our society—the attempt to remove whole spheres of behavior from moral scrutiny and judgment. That point needs a complementary one: a number of activities once thought to be only private in their moral significance are now judged to be of public importance. For example, the common moral wisdom tells us—in a way it did not tell Mill's generation—that we have among other things: no right to pollute the water and the air; to knowingly procreate defective children or even to have too many healthy children; to utter slurs against females, ethnic, or racial groups; or to ignore the private domestic life of public officials. Family planning was, in the days of Margaret Sanger, an entirely public and proscribed matter. Then, with the triumph of the family planning movement, it became an issue of wholly private morality. With the perception of a world population explosion, it became once again a public matter. The frequenting of prostitutes was once legal in many places, and thought to be a concern of private morality only. Not many feminists, aware of the degradation of women that has been a part of prostitution, are likely to be impressed with a private-morality-consenting-adult rationale. They are hardly keen on pornography either, and for the same kind of reason.

If it is so hard to separate the private and the public, why does the idea continue to persist? One reason is that, on occasion, it can serve to buttress our personal predilections or ideologies. I know that I cannot make a good moral case to myself about why I continue to smoke in the face of all that distressing health evidence. Yet I do not have to try quite so hard when I can persuade myself that the issue is between myself and myself and is no one else's affair. (That others ordinarily believe it necessary to cite potential harm to others as the essence of their moral point against me only confirms the power of a minimalist ethic.) Think also how much more arduous it would be morally for the "pro-choice" group in the abortion debate to have to admit that abortion decisions are fully public in their direct implications, and then to be forced to make the case for the public benefits of abortion. The argument could perhaps be made in some cases—but it is much, much easier to relegate the whole issue to the private realm, where the standards of moral rigor are more accommodating.

There are other, less self-serving reasons for the persistence of the distinction. We need some language and concepts for finding a limit to the right of the government, or the populace, to intervene in our lives. That was Mill's concern and it is as legitimate now as it was in his day. In groping around for a solution, our legal system stumbled on a "right to privacy." That concept represents a latter-day reading of the Constitution, and has resisted efforts to give it a clear meaning. Even so, it has its heuristic uses and no better formulation has been proposed to get at some kinds of civil liberties issues. Yet to say that the concept is useful does not mean that we need to reify, as if it represented reality, a sharp distinction between private and public life. A loose, shifting, casual distinction, taken with a nice grain of salt, may be equally serviceable.

The problem we now face is twofold. Do those of us who want to protect civil liberties have the nerve to openly admit the possibility that our society is paying an increasingly high moral cost for isolating the "private" sphere from moral judgment? We have certainly gained a number of valuable civil liberties as a result. But there is growing evidence that the diffuse and general consequences of that gain have been as harmful as they have been beneficial—the multiple indignities of daily life in large cities, for example. Mill was prepared to recognize that a price could well be paid for the liberty he proposed. But without offering any specific evidence, he simply asserted that it was a price worth paying. We have less reason to remain confident about that equation. He was not speaking about the realities of his own society but projecting one yet to be. Not until our own day have we seen, in actuality, what he had in mind. We can thus make a far better judgment than was possible for him. My own observation, however, is that defenders of his "simple principle" in its revised and extended "minimalist ethic" form are resolutely unwilling to look some unsavory reality straight in the face.

If that were done, we would be driven to grapple with the need to set some limits on those liberties which, in balance, produce an intolerable level of moral nihilism and relativism as a cultural outcome. It is not, and ought not to be, just the Moral Majority that worries about violence and more-tolerant-than-thou sex on television; or about children neglected by parental quests for greater psychological fulfillment; or about casual stealing, cheating, lying, and consenting-adult infidelity; or about rising assault and murder rates. Whatever the gain to liberty of the private standards and dispositions that tacitly support those developments, they all point to the emergence of an intolerable society, destructive as much to private as to public life. Any society can survive some degree of those vices, but life becomes much more fragile, and human relationships much less secure, when they are pervasive and inescapable. A legitimate respect for civil liberties does not require foregoing standards by which to judge private behavior any more than respect for freedom of speech requires suspending judgment on the contents of free speech.

Mill's problem was to find a "limit" to "the legitimate interference of collective opinion with individual independence. . . ."[16] While our task may not exactly be the opposite, the weight of inquiry may now have to shift. What ought to be the limits of liberty, and how can we identify those points at which "collective opinion" ought to hold sway against claims of private moral autonomy? To even ask that question implies that we must be prepared once again to judge the private lives of others and the way they use their liberty, and our standards ought to be more demanding than those required by a minimalist ethic.

Why should we believe that the sum total of private, self-interested acts that do no ostensible harm to others will add up to a favorable societal outcome? Those who would be the first to declaim against a pure economic market economy, guided by an "invisible hand," seem quite willing to tolerate a moral market economy, as if the result in the moral realm will be more favorable than in the economic. (There is an equal irony on the other side, of course: those who rage against a government-controlled economy seem quite prepared to accept a government-controlled morality.) There is equally no reason to believe that the good of the individual is necessarily the good of society, as if any free act is, by virtue of its freedom alone, a social contribution. That is especially true if the good is defined simply as moral autonomy and, to make matters worse, is combined with a systematic agnosticism about the morally proper uses of that autonomy. We are then deterred from passing a moral judgment on our neighbor (which he may well need and deserve) and, still more, harmed in our capacity as a society to determine what individual virtues, dispositions, and behaviors we want to promote and publicly support. Under a minimalist ethic that discussion cannot even begin. It is ruled out in principle.

The strong tendency in our society to confuse legal standards with moral principles has become a major part of the problem. When it is assumed that, under the aegis of liberty, moral judgment cannot be passed on private life, then the only general moral norms become those supplied by the law. On occasion, to be sure, the law can be a powerful and positive moral educator. The civil rights legislation of the 1960s gradually served to change moral attitudes as well as specific discriminatory practices, whatever the local bitterness it occasioned at the time. But just as frequently a change in the law—particularly a change that sees inhibitory laws removed from the books—can suggest that the matter has been removed from the moral order as well.

The proper relationship between law and morality is an old and difficult question. Yet it can only be fully meaningful when there are some generally accepted moral standards against which the law can be measured. If that is too strong a statement, then there must at least be an expectation that explicit limits will be recognized within the private moral order; put in the starkest terms, that behavior not controlled by statute will be controlled or modulated by the power of public opinion. And by "public opinion" I mean the direct and strong moral judgment of others. If (as I believe) the law should be minimal in publicly enforcing moral standards, that ought not mean a parallel shrinking of the moral realm. But that is precisely the conclusion a minimalist ethic entails. By default, law is left as the only standard by which to measure and reliably control behavior. It should thus be no surprise that, when cries of moral decline are in the air, many will immediately rush to the law to fill the vacuum. What does a minimalist ethic offer in the place of law? Nothing, and that by definition.


## AN ANTIDOTE TO THE MINIMALIST ETHIC?


Is there an antidote to a minimalist ethic, one that could avoid the moral anemia and casual ethical relativism that is its inevitable outcome, but avoid as well a reactionary reimposition of restrictions on hard-won civil liberties? I am not at all certain, and finding one will not be easy. Mill could make a strong case for his "simple principle" in the relationship between the individual and the state because he could assume a relatively stable body of moral conviction below the surface. Can we make a similar assumption? I think we must. There are no new and better values on the moral horizon than those we already possess: liberty, justice, human dignity, charity, benevolence, and kindness, and that is not a full list. A minimalist ethic cannot endure a serious attempt to deploy not just liberty and justice but all those values. Nor could it survive a new willingness to pass public judgment on conduct that the law may and should still permit.

Civil tolerance is hardly tolerance at all if one moral choice is in principle as good as another. It can only make sense, and show its full strength, when there are standards against which to measure behavior. Then, within limits, we can allow others to speak and act as they see fit. But we owe it both to them and to morality to let them know when we think they are behaving badly, whether to themselves or to others. We do not have to ban tawdry television programs, or publications, or obnoxious viewpoints. We just bring to bear all the private and public opinion we can against them. Will that work? It had better, for the next step will be far worse, and there are already many who would have the law do what ought to be the work of morality.

## References

1. Gerald L. Klerman, "Psychotropic Hedonism vs. Pharmacological Calvinism," *Hastings Center Report* (September 1972), pp. 1–3.
2. John Stuart Mill, "On Liberty," in *John Stuart Mill: Selected Writings*, ed. Mary Warnock (New York: Meridian Books, 1962), p. 135.
3. Ibid.
4. *Ibid.*, p. 130.
5. *Ibid.*, p. 138.
6. *Ibid.*, p. 135.
7. *Ibid.*, p. 206.
8. *Ibid.*, p. 207.
9. Gerald Dworkin has pointed out to me that Mill did not consider moral condemnation, even of a very harsh kind, a form of doing harm to another. *Cf* the following passage from *On Liberty*: "There is a degree of folly, and a degree of what may be called (though the phrase is not unobjectionable) lowness or a deprivation of taste, which, though it cannot justify doing harm to the person who manifests it, renders him necessarily and properly a subject of distaste, or, in extreme cases, even of contempt..." *Ibid.* p. 207.
10. Anonymous, circa 1980.
11. Mill, p. 190.
12. *Ibid.*, p. 212.
13. *Ibid.*, p. 213.
14. *Ibid.*, p. 138.
15. *Ibid.*, p. 209.
16. *Ibid.*, p. 130.

# 4

## INDIVIDUAL GOOD AND COMMON GOOD: A COMMUNITARIAN APPROACH TO BIOETHICS

When the field of bioethics began to emerge in the late 1960s and early 1970s, one of the first questions to surface was that of its ethical foundation. The earlier, historical field of medical ethics rested either on a theological base, stemming from various religious perspectives, or, much further back in time, on the professional obligations of the physician to the patient and to the profession, embodied in what we think of as the Hippocratic tradition.

The new bioethics, however, needed to find a way to speak in a secular culture, drawing on nonreligious premises, and to encompass a far wider range of medical and biotechnology issues than that of the doctor-patient relationship. The question then became: what ought to be the foundational principles, premises, and perspectives of this new venture? Two answers were quickly forthcoming. One was that the ethical foundations of the field should not be idiosyncratic to its particular issues but should be understood simply as an arena for the application of more general ethical principles and analysis. The other was just the opposite: bioethics should have its own moral basis, suitable to its particular subject matter.

That debate sputtered out by the end of the 1970s, never formally resolved but de facto influenced by the growing number of philosophers drawn to bioethics and prone to import into it the modes of reasoning common to the moral philosophy of the era. Most textbooks and classroom readers in bioethics came to open with an introduction to philosophical ethics, which usually turned out to be an inventory of the familiar philosophical theories of utilitarianism, deontology, natural law thinking, and the like. The idea that there is distinctive biomedical ethic all but disappeared from the inventory.

Two important developments since that time bear on the foundations of bioethics. The first is a general decline of interest in foundational matters—even though, for those who remain interested, there have been new theoretical models added to the older ones, such as feminist and narrative ethics. By "foundational matters," I mean broadly comprehensive theories of a kind symbolized by the arguments between utilitarians and deontologists. There nonetheless remains, at a somewhat lower level, a lively interest in the place of rules and principles, the balancing of universality and contextuality, and the virtues pertinent to patient care.

Although textbooks and readers still have introductions to ethical theory, it is striking how the majority of articles selected for inclusion in the readers are in fact devoid of the direct employment of any of those theories. They may be there tacitly, but it is rare to find them openly used to solve ethical problems. An examination of, say, the case studies carried for over 30 years now in the *Hastings Center Report* reveals a similar phenomenon. In both instances, the main characteristic is the lack of a conspicuous theory. The articles and case studies are, in that respect, all over the place in their analysis, marked by many strengths and charms (if any good at all), but theory is rarely prominent. While "principlism" (the view that four moral principles—autonomy, non-maleficence, beneficence, and justice— are sufficient to deal with most moral problems in medicine) still raises its head now and then, its numerous critics have taken much of the wind out of its sails (Beauchamp and Childress 2001).

The second development is not unrelated to the first, but moves in a different direction. It might best be characterized as the almost complete triumph of liberal individualism in bioethics. I call this an ideology rather than a moral theory because it is a set of essentially political and social values brought into bioethics, not as formal theory but as a vital background constellation of values. If it does not function as a moral theory as philosophers have understood that concept, it is clearly present and pervasive as a litmus test of the acceptability of certain ideas and ways of framing issues. As a familiar constellation it encompasses a high place for autonomy, for biomedical progress with few constraints, for procedural rather than substantive solutions to controverted ethical problems, and for a strong antipathy to comprehensive notions of the human good.

As a practical matter, the triumph of liberal individualism has led to a systematic marginalization of religious and conservative perspectives, often treated with disdain and hostility; and it has brought to bioethics the cultural wars from which it had earlier been spared. Bioethicists are increasingly labeled as "liberal" or "conservative," and the nastiness and partisanship of the broader political scene has begun to make its appearance (though mainly from the conservative side; liberals seem too indifferent to conservatives to care what they say). It is exceedingly rare to find ethical conferences or symposia that are not dominated by one side or the other, usually unwittingly (our congenial crowd), but sometimes consciously.

Many liberals were distressed that a conservative, Leon R. Kass, was appointed in 2001 to direct President Bush's Council on Bioethics, and that most of the Council members were of a similar persuasion. But each of the three earlier national bioethics commissions had liberal directors and predominantly liberal members, though that had been hardly noticed in the press, much less complained about, presumably because it was taken for granted. As it turned out, the Bush Council showed far more ethical variety and lack of consensus in its work on cloning than had been true of any of the other commissions; more than lip service has been paid to diversity (President's Council on Bioethics 2002). I was not proud of my field when I heard the first question of a prominent science reporter who called me in the summer of 2001 about the stem cell debate. "Why is it," she asked, "that everyone in bioethics is in lock step on stem cells?" A good question, to which I had no ready answer—at least none I was prepared to be quoted on.

I have tried to briefly lay out this historical background in order to set the stage for the two central points I want to make in this paper. The first is the contention that bioethics needs no formal foundations, if for no other reason than that it is, and ought to be, an interdisciplinary field, drawing upon many disciplines for its intellectual resources. No one discipline, whatever its foundation, can claim a privileged place. Of course, it is the lack of formal foundations that dooms interdisciplinary fields to the frowns of disciplinary purists, but that can be survived if some other traits are in place. The traits I believe are most important for bioethical inquiry are, on the one hand, determining the right set of questions to ask and issues to pursue; and, on the other, pursuing them with rationality, imagination, and insight. If that is done, people will listen and progress can be made.

My second contention is that liberal individualism needs a strong competitive voice, one that can be found in communitarianism. In addition to fomenting cultural wars, liberal individualism does not have the intellectual strength or penetration to deal effectively with the most important bioethical issues. Its "thin theory" of the good is a thin gruel for the future of bioethics.


ASKING THE RIGHT QUESTIONS


Contemporary bioethics took its rise from the advances in biomedical knowledge and technological innovation that marked the postwar years and that showed the inadequacy of the older medical ethics to encompass the new issues.

I have found it helpful to categorize the issues into three parts, reflecting the impact of the new developments. Each category suggests some fundamental questions for bioethics.

First, scientific knowledge and its practical applications have forced a change in our vision of the goals and purposes in medicine, not simply moving from care to cure, and from palliation to the saving of life, but also showing the possibility of using medical knowledge and techniques only indirectly related, if at all, to the preservation of health traditionally understood; and, at the outer edge, bringing the possibility of an enhancement of human nature and traits into view. That has left us with the question: what are the proper goals and uses of medicine?

Second, scientific knowledge and its applications have led us to reexamine the meaning of health. As a concept, "health" has always had a descriptive component, referring to various biological characteristics of the body and mind and the pathologies that can affect them, and a normative component, referring to the human desire for good health and the related fear of illness and disease. While it would be stretching things to say that health has been redefined recently (debates about its meaning are old and well developed), it does seem evident that the practical standards for what counts as good health, and the attendant expectations for it, have considerably escalated of late.

What was tolerable health earlier—or if intolerable, then fatalistically accepted—is increasingly often now rejected. Why should we suffer from old age, or cancer, or heart disease, or simply a less than perfect face? If research can be brought to bear on what ails us, or even just displeases us, then it ought to be pursued; and, best of all, past research success is taken to guarantee future success (exactly the opposite of the Security and Exchange Commission's required warning on the purchase of stocks and bonds). Since the reality of, and expectations about, health are a significant determinant of our overall sense of well-being, we are then left with the question: what are realistic expectations for our health and what kind of research should we support to achieve it?

Third, the technological developments have led us to what seems to me the most important matter of all: we have been led to reconsider, in the light of biomedical progress, what it means to live a life and to think about the nature of our human nature. Effective contraception has helped change the role of women, the procreation of children, and the significance of sexuality. Advances in the health of the elderly have meant changes in the place of old age in the individual life cycle (and what counts as "old") and in the place of the elderly in our social order. Genetic technologies open up new prospects for choosing the traits of our children, and thus affect both the parent-child relationship and the meaning of parenthood. What do we want to make of ourselves as human beings, and what kinds of lives ought we aspire to live?

I don't mean to suggest here that biomedical developments will be the sole determinants of how we may shape our ideas of medicine, health, and the ordering of our lives. Not only will those three categories interact with and affect each other, but they will also take place in the context of developments in information theory, environmental trends, bioterrorism and new natural pathogens, economic and urban life, and so on. Predicting the outcome of so complex a mix is next to impossible, and predicting the mix of moral, social, and political values that will animate them is no less difficult.

At the same time, it is not a threat to liberty to say that liberal individualism is poorly equipped to help us as human communities develop the moral perspectives to deal with the resulting complexity. Liberal individualism's greatest weakness is what is often thought its greatest strength: eschewing a public pursuit of comprehensive ways of understanding the human good and its future. But it takes an act of arbitrary imagination to see how the principle of autonomy, at the core of individualism, or that of market values as its ideological conservative twin, can provide any helpful guidance. Only if one believes in some version of an "invisible hand" shaping our individual goods into a common good, can that view be made plausible. The inescapable reality of the kinds of changes that biomedical progress introduce is that they affect our collective lives, our social and educational and political institutions, as well as those tacitly shared values that push our culture one way or the other.

As an individual, I need to make choices about how I will respond to those changes. But more important, *we* have to make political and social decisions about which choices will, and will not, be good for us as a community, and about the moral principles, rules, and virtues that ought to superintend the introduction of new technologies into the societal mainstream. Only if we believe that there will be no socially coercive or inadvertent culture-shaping consequences of present and forthcoming medical technologies can we deny the need to take common, and not just individual, responsibility for the deployment of a biomedicine that can change just about everything in our lives.


## ANALYTICAL VIRTUES

Bioethics can survive and even flourish in the absence of any formal or agreed-upon foundations. But it cannot do without a set of intellectual skills that will enable its leading questions to be approached in the richest and deepest way possible. My list of such skills would include rationality, imagination, and insight. Rarely will any one of them be adequate by itself; typically, each should come into play to enhance the possibility of a comprehensive judgment. Although I cannot do justice to each of those skills here, I will try to indicate a general direction for each of them.

## Rationality

While rationality is obviously important for those of us who think of ourselves as rational animals, it is a complex idea. Nothing is less helpful, I have observed, than moralistically urging people to be rational, as if that is the definitive answer to prejudice and wayward emotions. Rationality is often, of course, taken to be synonymous with the use of scientific knowledge (positivism, long moribund, never quite dies); or with being objective (more easily said than done, and almost always morally contestable); or with thinking consistently (as if that guarantees anything other than consistency); or with making logical moves from premises to conclusions (which anyone of ordinary intelligence can do).

The great problem in bioethics as elsewhere is getting the right premises and points of rational departure, and no one has ever proposed good procedures for doing that. In any case, it is by no means easy to think well, especially about those bioethical issues that are new and whose understanding cannot readily draw on accumulated human experience. Nor is it easy for any of us to see how our tacit political and social ideologies, lurking just below the surface, are pulling the strings of our "rational" thought. Being right and being rational are not necessarily synonymous. The careful and painstaking analysis characteristic of good philosophical work is no guarantee of reasonable outcomes, though it can certainly (and sometimes misleadingly) give that impression. Some very bad ideas have been elegantly argued. Nonetheless, with all those qualifications in mind, rationality remains important. Reason can, on occasion, cut through to some truths not reducible to the passions.

## Imagination

I reveal myself as a consequentialist by holding that any form of reasoning that does not reflect on the possible consequences and implications of a chain of reasoning is likely to be blind and illusory. Unfortunately, in bioethics it is often almost impossible to know the likely consequences of new technologies or even, at the clinical level, the likely medical outcome of many procedures with individual patients. That is where imagination comes in. We will have to project a future that is little grounded in past experience, or one in which the experience is too limited to be wholly reliable. Nonetheless, if we must act, we will have nothing better to go by. A comprehensive imagination is needed, beginning with the question of the kind of world we want to live in, and how the various imagined scenarios or alternatives will or won't contribute to that world. If a scenario will not contribute, then there should be a presumption against it, not to be overridden because some individuals, or some market considerations, might make it appear attractive. Knowledge of the outcomes of other technologies can be helpful in that exercise.

## Insight

In using the term *insight*, I have two dimensions in mind. One of them is self-insight, attempting to understand one's biases and proclivities and how either might interfere with good judgment by pushing our reasoning and emotions one way rather than another. The other dimension is that of insight into the context of, and cultural background of, the ethical problem. Where did it come from; how is context shaping it; what is its cultural meaning?

While careful personal observation can sometimes do the necessary work here, the social sciences provide a useful source of insight. A memorable instance of that for me, while working on the care of the dying, was an anthropological study of their care by medical residents. The study concluded that patients "died" for the residents when therapy was no longer effective. Death was a function of the available technology, not something that happened to bodies (Muller and Koenig 1988). That insight helped me to grasp the meaning of the "technological imperative" in a clearer way.

## A COMMUNITARIAN PREDILECTION

While I believe that liberal individualism is, in excessively large doses, a poor ideological base for bioethics, it is too much a valuable part of our culture to simply throw out in favor of an alternative ideology, even communitarianism. Instead, the challenge is to put them in tension with each other, understanding that on some occasions prudence and good judgment will decisively go one way or the other, and on other occasions there will be a compromise blend. The main point though is that communitarianism must be allowed to be a strong competitor—permitted, in fact, to make the opening bid in framing the issues. By the "opening bid" I simply mean that the *first* ethical question always to be raised should bear on the potential societal and cultural impact of a possible decision. While this approach is most evidently important with new technologies that can have major social implications (e.g., germ line therapy), it is no less applicable with the classical problems of individual patient choices and doctor-patient relationships. The fact that they present themselves as individual problems does not mean that they do not, in reality, have social implications. Those implications should always be sought out. Moreover, it is important to be able to interpret some principles assumed to be individualist in a communitarian way, as I will shortly try to show with "principlism."

Let me define what I mean by *communitarianism*. In fashioning a definition, the dominant image is one I take from ecology. The important question for ecologists when new species are introduced into an existing environment is not just how well they will flourish individually, but what they will do to the network of other species. Will they live in harmony with them, perhaps improving the whole ensemble, or will they prove destructive? Or will they perhaps do a little of both? The function of communitarianism is to force us to ask the ecology question, now brought into the realm of ethics. While I will use the example of new technologies and their dissemination as my main examples, a more extended analysis would encompass the full range of the ethical problems of contemporary medicine.

*Communitarianism*, as I construe the term, is meant to characterize a way of thinking about ethical problems. It is not meant to provide a formula or a set of rigid criteria for solving them. That is why I opened this essay with an emphasis on "analytical virtues" and on asking the right questions rather than on ethical theory as ordinarily understood. Communitarianism might best be understood as a stance or a way of framing issues. Thereafter, the analytic virtues I sketched above will come into play, offering no sure guide to good decisions, but instead the ingredients of a prudential richness that the mainline philosophical theories usually overshadow.

Here are some key categories to flesh out my understanding of communitarianism.

*Human nature.* Human beings are social animals. They always exist in a network of other people and within the social institutions and culture of their society.

*The public and the private.* No sharp distinction can be drawn between the public and private spheres. The private sphere is a fluctuating social construct with few if any intrinsic contents of its own. Although it is important that there be a private sphere, to protect against undue encroachments of public pressure and to acknowledge the diversity of human tastes, values, and ways of life, what counts as private will be a societal decision.

*The welfare of the whole.* Just as a sensitive ecologist will take the whole of a natural environment or landscape as the point of departure, so too a communitarian will begin with the welfare of a society as a whole as the analogous starting point—understanding "welfare" in the broadest sense, as encompassing the traditions, political institutions, characteristic practices and values, and culture commitments of a society.

*Human rights.* Every society needs a set of recognized individual rights, both negative and positive. They are imperative as a solid source of resistance to the power of government or public opinion when it goes awry. They also establish the moral standing of individuals, and thus serve to provide a sense of security in their thoughts and actions. At the same time, few human rights are unlimited. They can come in conflict with each other, requiring a choice or efforts at achieving some kind of reasonable balance. For example, some claims of reproductive rights, such as cloning, can threaten the right of a child to its own genetic future. A right to health care without limits in the face of scarce resources can threaten the health needs of others.

*Democratic participation.* When biomedical developments, theoretical or applied, are likely to affect the community as a whole, including its traditional values, then it is appropriate to initiate a community discussion of the human good, understood comprehensively. A society that avoids confronting the nature of the human good sets itself up to be influenced by the biomedical developments in ways beyond its control and direction. Every member of the community ought to have a part in these discussions, and be allowed to speak the language most congenial to their religious or secular values. The notion that "public reasons" only should count in the public square amounts to empowering groups whose culture easily make that possible at the expense of those which don't. In any case, wholly sectarian positions, though they should have an accepted place in democratic decision-making, are not likely to be efficacious in pluralistic societies.

*Individual good and common good.* The relationship between individual good and common good is an old issue. When analyzing the introduction of new technologies or the deployment of old ones, a communitarian predilection will require that the very first questions be asked from a communitarian perspective. What will the technology mean for all of us together? The next questions will address what the technology's meaning for individuals will be, and whether (1) the technology is sufficiently compatible with the common good to permit its use, and (2) if the technology is not wholly compatible, whether it should nonetheless be permitted on the grounds that a good society may on occasion permit potential harms to itself in the name of accommodating the special needs of some of its citizens.

Such an approach to biomedical technology would effectively turn upside down the working presumption of liberal individualism when evaluating technology. That presumption can be formulated as a general if not always articulated rule: if a new technology is desired by some individuals, they have a right to that technology unless hard evidence (not speculative possibilities) can be advanced showing that it will be harmful; since no such evidence can be advanced with technologies not yet deployed and in use, therefore the technology may be deployed.

This rule in effect means that the rest of us are held hostage by the desires of individuals and by the overwhelming bias of liberal individualism toward technology, which creates a presumption in its favor that is exceedingly difficult to combat. Such an argument has been used by some supporters of reproductive cloning, who invented heart-wringing scenarios designed to show that it would help some infertile people or help make up for the death of a loved one. Speculative objections were at first put aside, and it was only with the appearance of considerable evidence of harm to animals that even early proponents gave way. At no point, however, was a case advanced that cloning would make a contribution to the overall welfare of our society or any other—only the supposed good of some would-be parents was at stake, and not even their children.

## CONVERTING INDIVIDUALISTIC PRINCIPLES
## TO COMMUNITARIAN PRINCIPLES

I want to propose, in closing, that many well-accepted principles reflecting a commitment to liberal individualism can be converted into communitarian principles, and that they will be the richer for it. Principlism, for example, has been one of the most widely used methodological tools for the resolution of ethical dilemmas. It has been presented as a set of middle-level principles, of more utility than high-level principles, such as deontology and utilitarianism. While much criticized over the years, principlism has managed to survive, and it has been particularly popular with clinicians and others who want a relatively clear and simple way of thinking through ethical problems. Principlism has seemed to meet those needs, and it is usually presented as a non-ideological methodology.

In practice, however, principlism is an expression of liberal individualism. Its four principles are meant to cover the major ethical considerations that should bear on clinical and policymaking decisions. In reality, autonomy turns out to be king: all the other principles lead back to it, and the interpretation of the principles is classically liberal. Autonomy as interpreted by principlism enshrines the right to make one's own decisions, but assiduously avoids specifying a means of evaluating the ethical content of those decisions; nonmaleficence, aiming to protect patients from harm, is a variant of the autonomy principle, emphasizing negative liberty, the right of bodily noninterference; the point of justice as a principle is to ensure a sufficiently fair share of social and medical resources, such that individuals are free to make efficacious autonomous judgments in living their lives, unhampered by social inequities; and beneficence comes down to assisting people to be treated fairly and empowered to live their autonomous lives. It is no wonder that of all the principles, beneficence is the most neglected. For it to be taken with full seriousness would require coming to some judgment about what is actually beneficial to people. And that would mean crossing the brightest of all liberal lines, moving into the taboo territory of "the human good," about which too many bad things cannot be said.

Each of these principles admits of a communitarian translation. Autonomy should be broadened to encompass an analysis of what constitutes morally good and bad free choices. The claim that so-called private choices should be exempt from moral analysis is the death of ethics. Private choices can be right and wrong, good and bad, and at the least, we benefit from the moral counsel and judgment of our fellow citizens. How ought I to live? That question is an ancient part of ethics, not to be neutered by designations of private choice. Those private choices will determine in great part our view of how we ought to live together.

Non-maleficence should encompass an analysis of those harms other than physical that can be done to people, threats to their values and social relationships, for instance—that is, the making of judgments about what truly harms people in the broadest sense of "harms." Beneficence should include an effort, requiring community reflection and support, to determine just what constitutes the good of individuals, even if that means trespassing into the forbidden territory of comprehensive theories of the human good. Justice, finally, requires a judgment not only about what constitutes a fair distribution of health care resources but must—in the face of scarce resources—also determine just what constitutes appropriate resources, among those already available for distribution or those that could be created by research advances. If, for instance, we are interested in a fair allocation of future resources, what kind of a research agenda for what kind of medical progress would most promote it?

As these suggestions should make clear, I understand communitarianism to include a social rather than individual starting point for ethical analysis, but also a solid place for substantive reflection and judgment about ends and goals—and that is its greatest strength. Liberal individualism works overtime to avoid substantive analysis and judgment. Communitarianism goes in just the opposite direction, embracing the hardest and deepest questions about the right uses of medical knowledge and technology. Given their power to change the way we live our lives, and to understand our own nature, nothing else will suffice.

The greatest fear of liberal individualism is authoritarianism. But that fear, reasonable enough, fails to take account of the fact that the power of technology, and the profit to be made from it, can control and manipulate us even more effectively than authoritarianism. Moral dictators can be seen and overthrown, but technological repression steals up on us, visible but with an innocent countenance, and is just about impossible to overthrow, even as we see it doing its work on us. Liberal individualism makes this scenario more easily possible, and that is why it is not a tolerable guide to the sensible use of medical knowledge and technology.

It is just possible as well that a stronger place for communitarianism in our society will help to dampen the cultural war that has broken out in bioethics. A well-formulated communitarianism will not be indifferent to the rights and values of individuals; it will make room for them. In that respect, it need not worry political liberals as much as it does. A stronger appreciation of communitarianism could also hope to open up a stronger dialogue with conservative thought. Conservative thought is willing to take seriously the notion of a human good and of the need for substantive inquiry into the nature of good and evil in scientific progress and technological innovation. The liberal individualism of much contemporary bioethics needs to take seriously that way of thinking. Without it, bioethics risks being empty and leaving everyone else at the mercy of biomedical developments that will have their way with us. It should be the other way around.

## References

Beauchamp, T., and J. Childress. 2001. *Principles of biomedical ethics,* 5th ed. New York: Oxford Univ. Press.

Muller, J. H., and B. Koenig. 1988. On the boundary of life and death: The definition of dying by medical residents. In *Biomedicine examined,* ed. M. Lock and D. Gordon. Dordrecht: Kluwer Academic; 351–374.

President's Council on Bioethics. 2002. *Human cloning and human dignity.* New York: Public Affairs.

# 5

# THE WHO DEFINITION OF "HEALTH"

THERE is not much that can be called fun and games in medicine, perhaps because unlike other sports it is the only one in which everyone, participant and spectator, eventually gets killed playing. In the meantime, one of the grandest games is that version of king-of-the-hill where the aim of all players is to upset the World Health Organization (WHO) definition of "health." That definition, in case anyone could possibly forget it, is as follows: "Health is a state of complete physical, mental, and social well-being and not merely the absence of disease or infirmity." Fair game, indeed. Yet somehow, defying all comers, the WHO definition endures, though literally every other aspirant to the crown has managed to knock it off the hill at least once. One possible reason for its presence is that it provides such an irresistible straw man; few there are who can resist attacking it in the opening paragraphs of papers designed to move on to more profound reflections.

But there is another possible reason which deserves some exploration, however unsettling the implications. It may just be that the WHO definition has more than a grain of truth in it, of a kind which is as profoundly frustrating as it is enticingly attractive. At the very least it is a definition which implies that there is some intrinsic relationship between the good of the body and the good of the self. The attractiveness of this relationship is obvious: it thwarts any movement toward a dualism of self and body, a dualism which in any event immediately breaks down when one drops a brick on one's toe; and it impels the analyst to work toward a conception of health which in the end is resistant to clear and distinct categories, closer to the felt experience. All that, naturally, is very frustrating. It seems simply impossible to devise a concept of health which is rich enough to be nutritious and yet not so rich as to be indigestible.

One common objection to the WHO definition is, in effect, an assault upon any and all attempts to specify the meaning of very general concepts. Who can possibly define words as vague as "health," a venture as foolish as trying to define "peace," "justice," "happiness," and other systematically ambiguous notions? To this objection the "pragmatic" clinicians (as they often call themselves) add that, anyway, it is utterly unnecessary to know what "health" means in order to treat a patient running a high temperature. Not only that, it is also a harmful distraction to clutter medical judgment with philosophical puzzles.

Unfortunately for this line of argument, it is impossible to talk or think at all without employing general concepts; without them, cognition and language are impossible. More damagingly, it is rarely difficult to discover, with a bit of probing, that even the most "pragmatic" judgment (whatever *that* is) presupposes some general values and orientations, all of which can be translated into definitions of terms as general as "health" and "happiness." A failure to discern the operative underlying values, the conceptions of reality upon which they are based, and the definitions they entail, sets the stage for unexamined conduct and, beyond that, positive harm both to patients and to medicine in general.

But if these objections to any and all attempts to specify the meaning of "health" are common enough, the most specific complaint about the WHO definition is that its very generality, and particularly its association of health and general well-being as a positive ideal, has given rise to a variety of evils. Among them are the cultural tendency to define all social problems, from war to crime in the streets, as "health" problems; the blurring of lines of responsibility between and among the professions, and between the medical profession and the political order; the implicit denial of human freedom which results when failures to achieve social well-being are defined as forms of "sickness," somehow to be treated by medical means; and the general debasement of language which ensues upon the casual habit of labeling everyone from Adolf Hitler to student radicals to the brat next door as "sick." In short, the problem with the WHO definition is not that it represents an attempt to propose a general definition, but it is simply a bad one.

That is a valid line of objection, provided one can spell out in some detail just how the definition can or does entail some harmful consequences. Two lines of attack are possible against putatively hazardous social definitions of significant general concepts. One is by pointing out that the definition does not encompass all that a concept has commonly been taken to mean, either historically or at present, that it is a partial definition only. The task then is to come up with a fuller definition, one less subject to misuse. But there is still another way of objecting to socially significant definitions, and that is by pointing out some, baneful effects of definitions generally accepted as adequate. Many of the objections to the WHO definition fall in the latter category, building upon the important insight that definitions of crucially important terms with a wide public use have ethical, social, and political implications; defining general terms is not an abstract exercise but a way of shaping the world metaphysically and structuring the world politically.

Wittgenstein's aphorism, "don't look for the meaning, look for the use," is pertinent here. The ethical problem in defining the concept of "health" is to determine what the implications are of the various uses to which a concept of "health" can be put. We might well agree that there are some uses of "health" which will produce socially harmful results. To carry Wittgenstein a step further, "don't look for the uses, look for the abuses." We might, then, examine some of the real or possible abuses to which the WHO definition leads, recognizing all the while that what we may term an "abuse" will itself rest upon some perceived *positive* good or value.

## HISTORICAL ORIGIN & CONTEXT

Before that task is undertaken, however, it is helpful to understand the historical origin and social context of the WHO definition. If abuses of that definition have developed, their seeds may be looked for in its earliest manifestations.

The World Health Organization came into existence between 1946 and 1948 as one of the first major activities of the United Nations. As an outcome of earlier work, an Interim Commission to establish the WHO sponsored an International Health Conference in New York in June and July of 1946. At that Conference, representatives of 61 nations signed the Constitution of the WHO, the very first clause of which presented the now famous definition of "health." The animating spirit behind the formation of the WHO was the belief that the improvement of world health would make an important contribution to world peace; health and peace were seen as inseparable. Just why this belief gained ground is not clear from the historical record of the WHO. While there have been many historical explanations of the origin of World War II, a lack of world health has not been prominent among them; nor, for that matter, did the early supporters of the WHO claim that the Second World War or any other war might have been averted had there been better health. More to the point, perhaps, was the conviction that health was intimately related to economic and cultural welfare; in turn, that welfare, so it was assumed, had a direct bearing on future peace. No less important was a fervent faith in the possibilities of medical science to achieve world health, enhanced by the development of powerful antibiotics and pesticides during the war.

A number of memorandums submitted to a spring 1946 Technical Preparatory Committee meeting of the WHO capture the flavor of the period. The Yugoslavian memorandum noted that "health is a prerequisite to freedom from want, to social security and happiness." France stated that "there cannot be any material security, social security, or well-being for individuals or nations without health... the full responsibility of a free man can only be assumed by healthy individuals... the spread of proper notions of hygiene among populations tends to improve the level of health and hence to increase their working power and raise their standard of living. ... " The United States contended that "international cooperation and joint action in the furtherance of all matters pertaining to health will raise the standards of living, will promote the freedom, the dignity, and the happiness of all peoples of the world."

In addition to those themes, perhaps the most significant initiative taken by the organizers of the WHO was to include mental health as part of its working definition. In its memorandum, Great Britain stated that "it should be clear that health includes mental health," but it was Dr. Brock Chisholm, soon to become the first director of the WHO, who personified what Dr. Chisholm himself called the "visionary" view of health. During the meeting of the Technical Preparatory Committee he argued that: "The world is sick and the ills are due to the perversion of man; his inability to live with himself. The microbe is not the enemy; science is sufficiently advanced to cope with it were it not for the barriers of superstition, ignorance, religious intolerance, misery and poverty. ... These psychological evils must be understood in order that a remedy might be prescribed, and the scope of the task before the Committee therefore knows no bounds."

In Dr. Chisholm's statement, put very succinctly, are all of those elements of the WHO definition which led eventually to its criticism: defining all the problems of the world as "sickness," affirming that science would be sufficient to cope with the causes of physical disease, asserting that only anachronistic attitudes stood in the way of a cure of both physical and psychological ills, and declaring that the cause of health can tolerate no limitations. To say that Dr. Chisholm's "vision" was grandiose is to understate the matter. Even allowing for hyperbole, it is clear that the stage was being set for a conception of "health" which would encompass literally every element and item of human happiness. One can hardly be surprised, given such a vision, that our ways of talking about "health" have become all but meaningless. Even though I believe the definition is not without its important insights, it is well to observe why, in part, we are so muddied at present about "health."

## HEALTH & HAPPINESS

Let us examine some of the principal objections to the WHO definition in more detail. One of them is that, by including the notion of "social well-being" under its rubric, it turns the enduring problem of human happiness into one more medical problem, to be dealt with by scientific means. That is surely an objectionable feature, if only because there exists no evidence whatever that medicine has anything more than a partial grasp of the sources of human misery. Despite Dr. Chisholm's optimism, medicine has not even found ways of dealing with more than a fraction of the whole range of physical diseases; campaigns, after all, are still being mounted against cancer and heart disease. Nor is there any special reason to think that future forays against those and other common diseases will bear rapid fruits. People will continue to die of disease for a long time to come, probably forever.

But perhaps, then, in the psychological and psychiatric sciences some progress has been made against what Dr. Chisholm called the "psychological ills," which lead to wars, hostility, and aggression. To be sure, there are many interesting psychological theories to be found about these "ills," and a few techniques which can, with some individuals, reduce or eliminate anti-social behavior. But so far as I can see, despite the mental health movement and the rise of the psychological sciences, war and human hostility are as much with us as ever. Quite apart from philosophical objections to the WHO definition, there was no empirical basis for the unbounded optimism which lay behind it at the time of its inception, and little has happened since to lend its limitless aspiration any firm support.

Common sense alone makes evident the fact that the absence of "disease or infirmity" by no means guarantees "social well-being." In one sense, those who drafted the WHO definition seem well aware of that. Isn't the whole point of their definition to show the inadequacy of negative definitions? But in another sense, it may be doubted that they really did grasp that point. For the third principle enunciated in the WHO Constitution says that, "the health of all peoples is fundamental to the attainment of peace and security. . . ." Why is it fundamental, at least to peace? The worst wars of the 20th century have been waged by countries with very high standards of health, by nations with superior life-expectancies for individuals and with comparatively low infant mortality rates. The greatest present threats to world peace come in great part (though not entirely) from developed countries, those which have combated disease and illness most effectively. There seems to be no historical correlation whatever between health and peace, and that is true even if one includes "mental health."

How are human beings to achieve happiness? That is the final and fundamental question. Obviously illness, whether mental or physical, makes happiness less possible in most cases. But that is only because they are only one symptom of a more basic restriction, that of human finitude, which sees infinite human desires constantly thwarted by the limitations of reality. "Complete" well-being might, conceivably, be attainable, but under one condition only: that people ceased expecting much from life. That does not seem about to happen. On the contrary, medical and psychological progress have been more than outstripped by rising demands and expectations. What is so odd about that, if it is indeed true that human desires are infinite? Whatever the answer to the question of human happiness, there is no particular reason to believe that medicine can do anything more than make a modest, finite contribution.

Another objection to the WHO definition is that, by implication, it makes the medical profession the gate-keeper for happiness and social well-being. Or if not exactly the gate-keeper (since political and economic support will be needed from sources other than medical), then the final magic-healer of human misery. Pushed far enough, the whole idea is absurd, and it is not necessary to believe that the organizers of the WHO would, if pressed, have been willing to go quite that far. But even if one pushes the pretension a little way, considerable fantasy results. The mental health movement is the best example, casting the psychological professional in the role of high priest.

At its humble best, that movement can do considerable good; people do suffer from psychological disabilities and there are some effective ways of helping them. But it would be sheer folly to believe that all, or even the most important, social evils stem from bad mental health: political injustice, economic scarcity, food shortages, unfavorable physical environments, have a far greater historical claim as sources of a failure to achieve "social well-being."[1] To retort that all or most of these troubles can, nonetheless, be seen finally as symptoms of bad mental health is, at best, self-serving and, at worst, just plain foolish.

A significant part of the objection that the WHO definition places, at least by implication, too much power and authority in the hands of the medical profession, need not be based on a fear of that power as such. There is no reason to think that the world would be any worse off if health professionals made all decisions than if any other group did; and no reason to think it would be any better off. That is not a very important point. More significant is that cultural development which, in its skepticism about "traditional" ways of solving social problems, would seek a technological and specifically a medical solution for human ills of all kinds. There is at least a hint in early WHO discussions that, since politicians and diplomats have failed in maintaining world peace, a more expert group should take over, armed with the scientific skills necessary to set things right; it is science which is best able to vanquish that old Enlightenment bogeyman, "superstition." More concretely, such an ideology has the practical effect of blurring the lines of appropriate authority and responsibility. If all problems—political, economic and social—reduce to matters of "health," then there ceases to be any ways to determine who should be responsible for what.

## THE TYRANNY OF HEALTH

The problem of responsibility has at least two faces. One is that of a tendency to turn all problems of "social well-being" over to the medical professional, most pronounced in the instance of the incarceration of a large group of criminals in mental institutions rather than prisons. The abuses, both medical and legal, of that practice are, fortunately, now beginning to receive the attention they deserve, even if little corrective action has yet been taken. (Counterbalancing that development, however, are others, where some are seeking more "effective" ways of bringing science to bear on criminal behavior.)

The other face of the problem of responsibility is that of the way in which those who are sick, or purportedly sick, are to be evaluated in terms of their freedom and responsibility. Siegler and Osmond elsewhere in this issue discuss the "sick role," a leading feature of which is the ascription of blamelessness, of nonresponsibility, to those who contract illness. There is no reason to object to this kind of ascription in many instances—one can hardly blame someone for contracting kidney disease—but, obviously enough, matters get out of hand when all physical, mental, and communal disorders are put under the heading of "sickness," and all sufferers (all of us, in the end) placed in the blameless "sick role." Not only are the concepts of "sickness" and "illness" drained of all content, it also becomes impossible to ascribe any freedom or responsibility to those caught up in the throes of sickness. The whole world is sick, and no one is responsible any longer for anything. That is determinism gone mad, a rather odd outcome of a development which began with attempts to bring unbenighted "reason" and free self-determination to bear for the release of the helpless captives of superstition and ignorance.

The final and most telling objection to the WHO definition has less to do with the definition itself than with one of its natural historical consequences. Thomas Szasz has been the most eloquent (and most single-minded) critic of that sleight-of-hand which has seen the concept of health moved from the medical to the moral arena. What can no longer be done in the name of "morality" can now be done in the name of "health": human beings labeled, incarcerated, and dismissed for their failure to toe the line of "normalcy" and "sanity."

At first glance, this analysis of the present situation might seem to be totally at odds with the tendency to put everyone in the blame-free "sick role." Actually, there is a fine, probably indistinguishable, line separating these two positions. For as soon as one treats all human disorders—war, crime, social unrest—as forms of illness, then one turns health into a normative concept, that which human beings must and ought to have if they are to live in peace with themselves and others. Health is no longer an optional matter, but the golden key to the relief of human misery. We *must* be well or we will all perish. "Health" can and must be imposed; there can be no room for the luxury of freedom when so much is at stake. Of course the matter is rarely put so bluntly, but it is to Szasz's great credit that he has discerned what actually happens when "health" is allowed to gain the cultural clout which morality once had. (That he carries the whole business too far in his embracing of the most extreme moral individualism is another story, which cannot be dealt with here.) Something is seriously amiss when the "right" to have healthy children is turned into a further right for children not to be born defective, and from there into an obligation not to bring unhealthy children into the world as a way of respecting the right of those children to health! Nor is everything altogether lucid when abortion decisions are made a matter of "medical judgment" (see *Roe vs. Wade*): when decisions to provide psychoactive drugs for the relief of the ordinary stress of living are defined as no less "medical judgment"; when patients are not allowed to die with dignity because of medical indications that they can, come what may, be kept alive; when prisoners, without their consent, are subjected to aversive conditioning to improve their mental health.

## ABUSES OF LANGUAGE

In running through the litany of criticisms which have been directed at the WHO definition of "health," and what seem to have been some of its long-term implications and consequences, I might well be accused of beating a dead horse. My only defense is to assert, first, that the spirit of the WHO definition is by no means dead either in medicine or society. In fact, because of the usual cultural lag which requires many years for new ideas to gain wide social currency, it is only now coming into its own on a broad scale. (Everyone now talks about everybody and everything, from Watergate to Billy Graham to trash in the streets, as "sick.") Second, I believe that we are now in the midst of a nascent (if not actual) crisis about how "health" ought properly to be understood, with much dependent upon what conception of health emerges in the near future.

If the ideology which underlies the WHO definition has proved to contain many muddled and hazardous ingredients, it is not at all evident what should take its place. The virtue of the WHO definition is that it tried to place health in the broadest human context. Yet the assumptions behind the main criticisms of

the WHO definition seem perfectly valid. Those assumptions can be characterized as follows: 1) health is only a part of life, and the achievement of health only
a part of the achievement of happiness; 2) medicine's role, however important,
is limited; it can neither solve nor even cope with the great majority of social,
political, and cultural problems; 3) human freedom and responsibility must be
recognized, and any tendency to place all deviant, devilish, or displeasing human
beings into the blameless sick-role must be resisted; 4) while it is good for human
beings to be healthy, medicine is not morality; except in very limited contexts
(plagues and epidemics) "medical judgment" should not be allowed to become
moral judgment; to be healthy is not to be righteous; 5) it is important to keep
clear and distinct the different roles of different professions, with a clearly circumscribed role for medicine, limited to those domains of life where the contribution of medicine is appropriate. Medicine can save some lives; it cannot save
the life of society.

These assumptions, and the criticisms of the WHO definition which spring
from them, have some important implications for the use of the words "health,"
"illness," "sick," and the like. It will be counted an abuse of language if the word
"sick" is applied to all individual and communal problems, if all unacceptable
conduct is spoken of in the language of medical pathologies, if moral issues
and moral judgments are translated into the language of "health," if the lines of
authority, responsibility, and expertise arc so blurred that the health profession is
allowed to pre-empt the rights and responsibilities of others by re-defining them
in its own professional language.

Abuses of that kind have no possibility of being curbed in the absence of
a definition of health which does not contain some intrinsic elements of limitation—that is, unless there is a definition which, when abused, is self-evidently
*seen* as abused by those who know what health means. Unfortunately, it is in the
nature of general definitions that they do not circumscribe their own meaning (or
even explain it) and contain no built-in safeguards against misuse, e.g., our "peace
with honor" in Southeast Asia—"peace," "honor"? Moreover, for a certain class of
concepts—peace, honor, happiness, for example—it is difficult to keep them free
in ordinary usage from a normative content. In our own usage, it would make no
sense to talk of them in a way which implied they are not desirable or are merely
neutral: by well-ingrained social custom (resting no doubt on some basic features
of human nature) health, peace, and happiness are both desired and desirable—
good. For those and other reasons, it is perfectly plausible to say the cultural task
of defining terms, and settling on appropriate and inappropriate usages, is far
more than a matter of getting our dictionary entries right. It is nothing less than
a way of deciding what should be valued, how life should be understood, and
what principles should guide individual and social conduct.

Health is not just a term to be defined. Intuitively, if we have lived at all, it is something we seek and value. We may not set the highest value on health—other goods may be valued as well—but it would strike me as incomprehensible should someone say that health was a matter of utter indifference to him; we would well doubt either his sanity or his maturity. The cultural problem, then, may be put this way. The acceptable range of uses of the term "health" should, at the minimum, capture the normative element in the concept as traditionally understood while, at the maximum, incorporate the insight (stemming from criticisms of the WHO definition) that the term "health" is abused if it becomes synonymous with virtue, social tranquility, and ultimate happiness. Since there are no instruction manuals available on how one would go about reaching a goal of that sort, I will offer no advice on the subject. I have the horrible suspicion, as a matter of fact, that people either have a decent intuitive sense on such matters (reflected in the way they use language) or they do not; and if they do not, little can be done to instruct them. One is left with the pious hope that, somehow, over a long period of time, things will change.

## IN DEFENSE OF WHO

Now that simply might be the end of the story, assuming some agreement can be reached that the WHO definition of "health" is plainly bad, full of snares, delusions, and false norms. But I am left uncomfortable with such a flat, simple conclusion. The nagging point about the definition is that, in badly put ways, it was probably on to something. It certainly recognized, however inchoately, that it is difficult to talk meaningfully of health solely in terms of "the absence of disease or infirmity." As a purely logical point, one must ask about what positive state of affairs disease and infirmity are an absence of—absent from what? One is left with the tautological proposition that health is the absence of non-health, a less than illuminating revelation. Could it not be said, though, that at least intuitively everyone knows what health is by means of the experiential contrast posed by states of illness and disease; that is, even if I cannot define health in any positive sense, I can surely know when I am sick (pain, high fever, etc.) and compare that condition with my previous states which contained no such conditions? Thus one could, in some recognizable sense, speak of illness as a deviation from a norm, even if it is not possible to specify that norm with any clarity.

But there are some problems with this approach, for all of its commonsense appeal. Sociologically, it is well known that what may be accounted sickness in one culture may not be so interpreted in another; one culture's (person's) deviation from the norm may not necessarily be another culture's (person's) deviation.

In this as in other matters, commonsense intuition may be nothing but a reflection of different cultural and personal evaluations. In addition, there can be and usually are serious disputes about how great a deviation from the (unspecified) norm is necessary before the terms "sickness" and "illness" become appropriate. Am I to be put in the sick role because of my nagging case of itching athlete's foot, or must my toes start dropping off before I can so qualify? All general concepts have their borderline cases, and normally they need pose no real problems for the applicability of the concepts for the run of instances. But where "health" and "illness" are concerned, the number of borderline cases can be enormous, affected by age, attitudinal and cultural factors. Worse still, the fact that people can be afflicted by disease (even fatally afflicted) well before the manifestation of any overt symptoms is enough to discredit the adequacy of intuitions based on how one happens to feel at any given moment.

A number of these problems might be resolved by distinguishing between health as a norm and as an ideal. As a norm, it could be possible to speak in terms of deviation from some statistical standards, particularly if these standards were couched not only in terms of organic function but also in terms of behavioral functioning. Thus someone would be called "healthy" if his heart, lungs, kidneys (etc.) functioned at a certain level of efficiency and efficacy, if he was not suffering physical pain, and if his body was free of those pathological conditions which even if undetected or undetectable could impair organic function and eventually cause pain. There could still be dispute about what should count as a "pathological" condition, but at least it would be possible to draw up a large checklist of items subject to "scientific measurement"; then, having gone through that checklist in a physical exam, and passing all the tests, one could be pronounced "healthy." Neat, clean, simple.

All of this might be possible in a static culture, which ours is not. The problem is that any notion of a statistical norm will be superintended by some kind of ideal. Why, in the first place, should anyone care at all how his organs are functioning, much less how well they do so? There must be some reason for that, a reason which goes beyond theoretical interest in statistical distributions. Could it possibly be because certain departures from the norm carry with them unpleasant states, which few are likely to call "good": pain, discrimination, unhappiness? I would guess so. In the second place, why should society have any interest whatever in the way the organs of its citizens function? There must also be some reason for that, very possibly the insight that the organ functioning of individuals has some aggregate social implications. In our culture at least (and in every other culture I have ever heard of) it is simply impossible, finally, to draw any sharp distinction between conceptions of the human good and what are accounted significant and negatively evaluated deviations from statistical norms.

That is the whole point of saying, in defense of the WHO definition of health, that it discerned the intimate connection between the good of the body and the good of the self, not only the individual self but the social community of selves. No individual and no society would (save for speculative, scientific reasons only) have any interest whatever in the condition of human organs and bodies were it not for the obvious fact that those conditions can have an enormous impact on the whole of human life. People do, it has been noticed, die; and they die because something has gone wrong with their bodies. This can be annoying, especially if one would, at the moment of death, prefer to be busy doing other things. Consider two commonplace occurrences. The first I have alluded to already: dropping a heavy brick on one's foot. So far as I know, there is no culture where the pain which that event occasions is considered a good in itself. Why is that? Because (I presume) the pain which results can not only make it difficult or impossible to walk for a time but also because the pain, if intense enough, makes it impossible to think about anything else (or think at all) or to relate to anything or anyone other than the pain. For a time, I am "not myself" and that simply because my body is making such excessive demands on my attention that nothing is possible to me except to howl. I cannot, in sum, dissociate my "body" from my "self" in that situation; my self is my body and my body is my pain.

The other occurrence is no less commonplace. It is the assertion the old often make to the young, however great the psychological, economic, or other miseries of the latter: "at least you've got your health." They are saying in so many words that, if one is healthy, then there is some room for hope, some possibility of human recovery; and even more they are saying that, without good health, nothing is possible, however favorable the other conditions of life may be. Again, it is impossible to dissociate good of body and good of self. Put more formally, if health is not a sufficient condition for happiness, it is a necessary condition. At that very fundamental level, then, any sharp distinction between the good of bodies and the good of persons dissolves.

Are we not forced, therefore, to say that, if the complete absence of health (i.e., death) means the complete absence of self, then any diminishment of health must represent, correspondingly, a diminishment of self? That does not follow, for unless a disease or infirmity is severe, it may represent only a minor annoyance, diminishing our selfhood not a whit. And while it will not do to be overly sentimental about such things, it is probably the case that disease or infirmity can, in some cases, increase one's sense of selfhood (which is no reason to urge disease upon people for its possibly psychological benefits). The frequent reports of those who have recovered from a serious illness that it made them appreciate life in a far more intense way than they previously had are not to be dismissed (though one wishes an easier way could be found).

## MODEST CONCLUSIONS

Two conclusions may be drawn. The first is that some minimal level of health is necessary if there is to be any possibility of human happiness. Only in exceptional circumstances can the good of self be long maintained in the absence of the good of the body. The second conclusion, however, is that one can be healthy without being in a state of "complete physical, mental, and social well-being." That conclusion can be justified in two ways: (a) because some degree of disease and infirmity is perfectly compatible with mental and social well-being; and (b) because it is doubtful that there ever was, or ever could be, more than a transient state of "complete physical, mental, and social well-being," for individuals or societies; that's just not the way life is or could be. Its attractiveness as an ideal is vitiated by its practical impossibility of realization. Worse than that, it positively misleads, for health becomes a goal of such all-consuming importance that it simply begs to be thwarted in its realization. The demands which the word "complete" entail set the stage for the worst false consciousness of all: the demand that life deliver perfection. Practically speaking, this demand has led, in the field of health, to a constant escalation of expectation and requirement, never ending, never satisfied.

What, then, would be a good definition of "health"? I was afraid someone was going to ask me that question. I suggest we settle on the following: "health is a state of physical well-being." That state need not be "complete," but it must be at least adequate, i.e., without significant impairment of function. It also need not encompass "mental" well-being; one can be healthy yet anxious, well yet depressed. And it surely ought not to encompass "social well-being," except insofar as that well-being will be impaired by the presence of large-scale, serious physical infirmities. Of course my definition is vague, but it would take some very fancy semantic footwork for it to be socially misused; that brat next door could not be called "sick" except when he is running a fever. This definition would not, though, preclude all social use of the language of "pathology" for other than physical disease. The image of a physically well body is a powerful one and, used carefully, it can be suggestive of the kind of wholeness and adequacy of function one might hope to see in other areas of life.

# 6

## END-OF-LIFE CARE: A PHILOSOPHICAL OR MANAGEMENT PROBLEM?

Early in 1970, just as we were organizing the Hastings Center, we had to decide which issues on a long menu of possibilities should receive our early attention. At the top of our list was end-of-life care. Complaints about care for the dying had mounted during the 1960s, fueled by technological progress in sustaining life, by too many patients abandoned by physicians as they lay dying, by a lack of patient choice on how their lives should end, and by woefully inadequate pain management. After a few years of study, the care of the dying seemed to admit of a solution: giving patients more choice by the use of living wills or appointment of a surrogate, improving the training of physicians to better deal with death and discussion with patients, and creating a hospice movement and greatly enhanced palliative care.

But here we are four decades later, not quite back where we started, but much less far along than we had naively thought possible. While I have varied the titles a bit, I have written at least four articles over the decades that have simply reworked a persistent question on end-of-life care: why has it been so hard? I have chewed on that bone and so have many others. To be sure, progress has been made. Probably close to 25% of adult Americans have a living will and/or have appointed a surrogate. Over 900,000 of us die each year in the care of a hospice program. Palliative care is now a medical specialty and doctors receive a better education in communicating with patients.

Still, the problem persists. Why is that? Is it possible to imagine actually solving it? And just what kind of problem is it anyway? That last question is the one I want to focus on. The de facto answer to that question, in the American can-do mode, is that it is a management and education issue, that is, one in which better medical techniques and health care policies together with improved public and professional education can manage the need. While that approach is eminently sensible and necessary, it is unlikely to work to the fullest extent necessary. It is inherently limited in its possibilities. Many people will continue to die in ways bad for themselves and their families.

For a full solution, good care for the dying now needs to be seen as a problem that needs a parallel public and professional discussion at what I will loosely call the philosophical level. Two basic questions need to be put on the table. One of them is what we take to be the place of death in human life, and the other, that of the place of death in medicine and health care. If one pushes far enough with the management and education strategy, asking why that has not been sufficient, I believe one will inevitably run into those two philosophical questions.

One will no less run into considerable resistance in confronting them. Not only are they hard questions to answer, if pushed far enough the likely answers imply a revolution in our medical thinking, clinical practice, and public policy. To make that case plausible I want first to examine the present management and education strategies to show how they fall short and must, almost certainly, do so. Each embodies some important obstacles to good end-of-life care. Then I will lay out the rudiments of a strategy that combines a management and philosophical approach. The management and education strategies can be grouped under three groups of obstacles: medical and health policy, physician and hospital practices, and patient and family values.

Modern medicine has on offer what I call the great trade-off: if you put your life in our hands, we will (for the most part) save you from a quick death by a heart attack or infectious disease thus allowing you to contract later in life a number of chronic diseases that will allow (or force) you to die much more slowly. Had you contracted a lethally infectious disease 150 years ago and survived, you would be back in good health, but with a much shorter life span thereafter in those days. With chronic disease you will most likely have a much longer life, but spend a significant portion of your old age in poor health, inexorably declining.

Is that a good bargain? Most of us seem to think so. We prefer to die old rather than young, our children to make it out of childhood and live a long life, and to take our chances with chronic disease. But it is also a costly bargain, economically, socially, and for many of us, personally as well. Economically, the cost of chronic disease is an enormous part of our health care spending, with some 20% of those with chronic disease accounting for an estimated 64% of our annual health care costs.[1] Some 25% of Medicare costs go to 6% of beneficiaries in the last year of life. Heart disease (27%) and cancer (23%) are the leading causes of death followed by stroke (6%), lower respiratory illness (5%), and Alzheimer's (3%).[2] "These data suggest," a comprehensive study concluded, "that virtually all Americans will have a substantial period of serious illness and disability at some point before death."[3]

In sum, medicine can offer no cures for chronic diseases, only the capacity to keep us alive longer with one or more of them. It is possible to save a person's life from cancer at 65, putting them on drugs and monitoring them thereafter, to save them from heart disease at 75 (with still more drugs to keep them going), and then to draw out such at life at 85 with Alzheimer's disease. As the Congressional Budget Office determined in 2008, "Examples of new treatments for which long-term savings have been demonstrated are few...improvement in mortality that decreases mortality...paradoxically increases overall spending on health care."[4]

Quite apart from the cost and prevalence of chronic disease, the care of patients with them poses a number of clinical difficulties for end-of-life care. Three of them stand out. The first is that, as Joanne Lynn has shown, the downward trajectory toward death varies from one disease to another.[5] Cancer is the most predictable (and a major reason it dominates hospice care), with a slow downward slope but very rapid toward the end. Heart disease sees a steady decline toward death as well but marked by unpredictable spikes of improvement along the way. Alzheimer's and frailty have a long, slow, and steady downward slope.

The second difficulty is that the variety of trajectories makes it difficult to determine exactly when the line between living and dying has been crossed, and made all the harder by the possibility that one or more aggressive technological interventions can extend life a few days, or even weeks, longer—and is further complicated by multi-organ failure, with different options of treatments for different organs, some failing with different degrees of damage and with speeds of decline.

The third clinical difficulty is that a high percentage of patients will end up in a hospital as their health deteriorates. The culture and ethos of hospitals is biased toward aggressive care and, when the first and second features are present, that bias works against good end-of-life care. By the word "good," I mean the control of pain, the avoidance of unnecessary diagnostic and treatment procedures, well-coordinated care, and family satisfaction.

How are most people with chronic disease kept alive? New and old technologies—drugs, devices, and high-technology hospital and ICU time—is the answer. Medical research, regularly touted as the royal road to cost control, has just the opposite results, producing those technologies that can extend our dying from disease but not cure them.[6] The estimates of technology-induced annual cost escalation range from 40%–60%, with 50% the most common.[7] A variety of efforts over the years to control technology costs have, with one exception, failed. The exception was in the mid-1990s, when managed care succeeded in flattening the upward cost curve for a couple of years. It was, unfortunately, a short-lived success, done in by physician and patient complaints. Certificate-of-need programs at the state level, meant to curb excessive hospital growth and expensive technologies, met a similar fate. Formulas established in the Medicare program to cut physician reimbursement were regularly over-ruled by Congress (which had put them in place).

Most important, the use of new technologies or intensified use of old ones on the critically ill has been driven by an overpowering set of incentives. They include fee-for-service medicine, paying physicians for the piecemeal use of technology, the training and acculturation of doctors aggressively to use technology, fear of malpractice suits, often excessive patient demands and expectations, direct-to-consumer advertising, constant industry advertising to physicians backed by pharmaceutical detail men going straight to doctors, and a media that dotes on medical breakthroughs and "promising" research.[8] Persistently rejected have been the means used by European health care systems to control costs: price controls, hospital and national budgets, control of the introduction of new technologies, and much lower salaries and fees for health care workers.

Will the reforms put in place by the reform legislation—such as comparative effectiveness research, an Independent Medicare Advisory Board, and cutbacks of physician reimbursement—make a difference? They may, but with many of them being put in place later in the decade, it will be years before we know answer to that question. Whether they will make a difference in end-of-life care is no less unknown. One hopeful sign is that although the reform legislation did not directly embody a provision from the earlier House bill to pay for physician consultations for Medicare beneficiaries, it did put provisions into palliative care provisions to do just that.[9]

But cost control will be a daunting task. The combination of a growing number of elderly entering the Medicare program over the next two decades, an endless stream of new or updated technologies to treat chronic disease, most of them expensive, and likely high expectations of the retiring baby boomers about getting the best and latest, will put new and unprecedented pressure on the health care system. Much of this noxious combination will be played out with end-of-life care, particularly at the intersection of critical illness and the possibility, but not certainty of death.

I have so far emphasized features pertinent to care of the dying at what can be called the macro-level of our health care system and how it shapes incentives to practice a particular kind of medicine—and creating obstacles willy-nilly to good end-of-life care. When one looks more closely at the clinical level, and particularly at patients, the doctor-patient relationship, and hospitals and the use of technologies, the scope of the obstacles is increased.

American patients appear to have a greater belief in, and desire for, medical technology than is the case in other countries.[10] One international survey, for instance, revealed that some 66% of Americans were "very interested" in new medical discoveries compared with a European average of 44%. Some 34% believe that medicine can cure any illness if they have access to the most advanced technology and treatment compared with only 27% of Canadians and 11% of Germans. The authors of the study judged that this high level of belief in technology will make it hard for Medicare to "restrain future Medicare expenditures for those technologies."[11] I would add to that judgment one likely explanation of a common lament of physicians, that of excessive patient expectations that medicine can do miracles, including saving their lives against all odds.

Some recent social science research has revealed a rise in the number of medical interventions that aim to prolong the life of the elderly. As the risk of cardiac interventions decline, "older individuals, their families and physicians feel able to justify their use even when they believe the benefit to be gained is negligible."[12] A study of HMOs and medical technology found that it was exceedingly difficult to control the adoption of new technologies because of hospital pressures to have them for competitive benefits, physician pressures to have the latest and the best, and lack of evidence on their value (the lack of evidence serving, ironically, to make them harder to resist).[13]

The availability of the new and improved technologies—some of whose cost must be amortized (but is a money machine) and which the culture of medical specialties is honed to use—underscores a point made above about patient care: the improvements in medical technologies increase the difficulty of finding a bright line between living and dying. They both invite aggressive efforts to keep critically ill patients alive from the physician side and encourage hopes, often false, from the patient side.

The much-lamented failure of coordinated care for the acutely ill is no help either, and that failure is built on the back of woefully inadequate primary care before people become sick. There has been a well-publicized decline in a solid doctor-patient relationship combined with poor continuity and integration of care in moving patients from the primary care to the critical care level. There has been agreement for years about the importance of end-of-life discussions between doctors and patients either while patients are still in good health or early on with the advent of serious illness. The decline in primary care, and the overwork of physicians who still practice it, makes such discussions increasingly less possible. And then, when a patient is critically ill with one or more chronic diseases, the care is likely to be uncoordinated and erratic, juggled around by specialists who may, or may not, be adequately communicating with each other. Decisions about desired and appropriate end-of-life care too often take place in a rushed, emotion-charged atmosphere. Even when there has been careful early discussion with a primary care physician, there is no good assurance that decisions earlier reached will be known or seriously considered by hospital physicians, that more complex choices than earlier envisioned will not present themselves, and that patients and their families will not have second thoughts about desired care.

In any event, ambivalence and anguish can mark even the best efforts to deal with the complexities of many deaths. Three stories illustrate some of them.

In one of the stories, about a man with kidney cancer, he and his wife fought against a disease that at first looked treatable but then began metastasizing to the point of exceedingly poor odds "at the far end of the bell curve," as his physician put it. The article's title catches the ambivalence felt in dealing with it, "End of Life Warning at $618,616 Makes Me Wonder If It Was Worth it."[14] They did everything possible to beat those poor odds, bearing a great deal of misery and disappointment along the way. In the end, all that effort was a failure. Or was it? The patient's wife said afterwards, "Would I do it all again? Absolutely. I couldn't not do it again." It gave her, she said, 17 extra months with her husband that she would otherwise not have had. But, she also said, had her husband known about the total costs, he would have stopped aggressive treatment much earlier.

David Rieff, the son of writer Susan Sontag, wrote a moving book about his mother's death from cancer, noteworthy because she was prepared to go to any financial length and physical suffering to fight the cancer that killed her, and she did.[15] Her son was put in the difficult position of supporting what he knew to be her near-illusory hopes.

Another story, by Kay Butler, related the struggle of a woman to have her stroke-damaged husband's pacemaker disconnected against the opposition of his cardiologist. "The pacemaker," his daughter said, "brought my parents two years of limbo, two of purgatory, and two of hell."[16] Eventually she and her mother succeeded, but even so she was torn at the end: "I felt as if I were signing on as his executioner."

Nothing I have said so far is meant to suggest that managerial and educational efforts have failed, or that further progress is not possible. Improvements in palliative care, in expanding the scope of hospice beyond the care of cancer patients (where it has been strongest), in a gradual increase of those with advance directives, and improved physician education are all hopeful signs. There is also by now good evidence that, with solid and candid information about their medical prognosis, knowledge of their options, and continuing doctor-patient discussion encompassing patients and families, patients are less likely to choose aggressive treatment. In short, there are some good strategies available and with evidence to back them up. But at the present pace of progress (it has taken over 40 years to get this far), that still leaves the prospect that thousands of patients will, as matters now stand and for the foreseeable future, die unnecessarily poor deaths.

Part of the reason for my pessimism is simply that care of the dying concentrates a wide range of variables, requiring the practice of good medicine in the hands of physicians well educated about, and sensitive to, the needs of the dying (and the former does not entail the latter), a good social and cultural setting for dying, and thoughtful and well-informed patients with hardly less required for their families and surrogates. As with the care of those suffering from chronic diseases that are now the leading cause of death, many things must come together for a satisfactory outcome.

Yet I think that the most important obstacle to good care of the dying lies at what I call the philosophical level. That problem is most pronounced in a fundamental tension within the modern medical enterprise. The essence of that tension is, on the one hand, that of the necessity of accepting death as an inevitable part of human life in order to make dying a tolerable experience—every physician must understand that every one of his patients will eventually die, sooner or later, and either on his own watch or that of some other physician. Medicine has known that ancient truth since the beginning, but has of late tried to ignore it. That result is a confident and ambitious science-oriented medicine that has, at least since WWII, treated death as an enemy that can be beaten, not all at once but one lethal disease at a time.

Ever since Richard Nixon in 1970 all but declared "war" on cancer—building on the ever optimistic budget and expanding momentum of the National Institutes of Health—American medicine in its research arm has treated death as a contingent human reality. William Haseltine, the CEO of Human Genome Sciences, once declared that "death is nothing but a preventable disease."[17] That was an excessive statement, but I doubt that any director of the NIH would, in testifying before Congress on its annual appropriation, identify any lethal disease as unconquerable. The research arm of medicine has eschewed fatalism in the struggle against death, and has recruited clinicians, legislators, the media, and the public to join in the fight.

If that is a correct perception, then the greatest enemy of a good death is the medical enterprise itself, powerfully inculcating the values of a utopian project against mortality, one that spills over into clinical practice. Patients have been culturally tutored to expect medical miracles, and the public has been fed a steady diet of hope and expectation. Recall the Human Genome Project, touted to get to the bottom of all disease and open the door to certain cure, and the fanfare that accompanied the research on embryonic stem cells, sure to save millions of lives, and the by-now almost annual ritual announcement of a soon-to-be-discovered cure for cancer. What my psychologist wife has called the "pathologies of hope" has been a leading feature of American medical research advocacy and ready media amplification, and is thus a leading cause of an intensification of patient expectations. The research war against death has come to imitate the trench warfare of WWI, with millions of lives lost in battles that gained only small amounts of land and that rarely led to decisive victories. Death from infectious disease has not gone away either as was once predicted and the success of research in finding a treatment for HIV disease is one of the few victories of recent medical progress.

Should we give up hope on research? Not at all, but yes on the hope it will lower costs; yet some realism is in order. Part of the realism should come with a sober acceptance of what I believe to be a fact: the chronic diseases of aging have run up against the reality of human aging and decline, built into all biological creatures. Considerable progress has been made against that reality, but future progress is likely to be harder not easier, as now seems to be the trend with a recent leveling off of average life expectancy.

A British clinician, Iona Heath, has offered another dose of realism: "All clinicians caring for older people have the experience of treating one disease process, only for another to take its place, and the more diseases that coexist, the greater the hazards of overtreatment and polypharmacy. ... When one cause of death is curtailed, others must inevitably come forward to fill the gap. Everyone is obliged to die of something."[18]

In the absence of that kind of sobriety—to which the research enterprise is allergic—we should hardly be surprised if the ancient hope that physicians have been taught to inspire in patients has been amplified by the hope inspired by a research imperative. The premise of that imperative is that medical progress, particularly against death, is a moral obligation: push on and don't give up hope. The combination of an ancient tradition of inspiring hope in patients, now joining hands with the modern moral obligation of inspiring hope in the onward progress of medicine, make for the last and greatest obstacle to good end of life care.

The message is that life should not end, and a future medicine, armed with more and better research and improved clinical skills, will eventually win the day. A notably interesting medical anthropology study some years ago of physician practices in the care of the dying found that "the patient is not even defined as dying until the clinicians determine that there are no further interventions they can make that will improve the patient's condition. Acknowledgment of a patient's dying status may not be made until death is imminent or, in some cases, has already occurred."[19] In other words, death is not something that happens to the body but is simply a function of available technology's capacity to hold it at bay. Between an attitude of that kind among physicians and reluctance as well on their part to discuss death, and patient and family resistance to conceding death is on its way, it is hardly any wonder that a chronic problem for hospice care is that of patients coming to it much later than they should.

I have dug a deep hole for end-of-life care to climb out of, a mixture of (a) obstacles at the level of management of the care of the dying and the education of physicians and patients, and (b) the obstacles created by a progress-driven, technologically infatuated medicine that has turned its face against dying and relentlessly scales the ladders of the trenches to face the enemy. Nor should I fail to mention that if the biology of human life moves us inevitably toward death, it no less moves us to resist it. A fundamental conflict is built into our biology, and not easily put aside in the care of the dying. A divided heart and mind goes with the territory, and rightly so.

How can we dig ourselves out of the hole? It will probably never be wholly possible. With individual patients, there will almost always be some conflicting emotions and ambivalent judgments in their own minds, conflicting medical assessments among physicians, and conflicting cultural attitudes about the right balance between cure and care in health care. We are not likely, that is, to find a fully rational way—in the narrow sense of that term, that is, no untidy emotions, no lingering uncertainty, and no easy decision pathways—to overcome all the obstacles. But we can move the national and professional discussion along in a productive way.

I will not try here to offer some immediately useful practical ideas about moving along the present efforts. They are already plentiful and useful. Almost all of them over the years have come down to refining the three target areas initially discerned in the 1970s: increasing patient knowledge and options, improving physician education, and putting in place strong hospice and palliative care programs. That work is continuing and steadily improving.

But it will be no less necessary to find ways of stimulating on a parallel but ultimately converging track the kind of substantive, philosophical discussion about death in our lives and in health care that I have tried to outline. I have already provided one reason to do so: the philosophical issues have always been there, just below the surface, and good end-of-life care cannot be achieved unless they are taken on fully and deeply. The other reason is that end-of-life care epitomizes in a striking way the larger problem of American medicine and health care. That problem is simply that we have a health care system that is too costly; too unwilling under the sway of market freedom to live with system-wide budgets; too dominated by an endless progress and innovation model of medicine; too careless about assessing the effectiveness of medical technologies and practice patterns; too resistant to thinking about death; and too reluctant to consider the possibility that the end-of-life debate has invited us to rethink the balance of care (once dominant) and cure (now dominant), applicable in most areas of health care.

Unless we change many of the underlying values of our health care system, much too readily taken for granted as sacred, we will have a system that is economically and humanly not sustainable over the long run, nor the intellectual resources to deal more effectively with the obstacles to the efficacious care of the dying. The two needs are inseparable.

Now let me confess, as a long-time veteran of writing upon this topic, that much of what I am saying here is not altogether fresh insight from me. But, having run into resistance, even indifference, I keep chewing on the bone. I have encountered three forms of resistance in trying to induce a wide discussion of what I see as the twin topics of death and medical progress. One of them is that for most people, it is self evident that death is an ultimate evil (unless one is here and now unbearable suffering and irreversible pain), and that medical progress is an unassailable good, the more the better. For them it is simply wrong to raise the topics. For others, their general agreement is that they are worth a discussion, but that assent is shadowed by a belief that neither the medical profession nor our society is up to and ready for that kind of discussion. It is too hard, too deep, and too subversive of deeply held convictions (even if maybe wrongheaded) to get us anywhere. And then there are those who believe that yes, these are worthy topics of consideration, but that it is too difficult in our pluralistic society, rent by value disagreements, to get very far with substantive discussions. It is safer and more productive to stay with procedural, educational, and organizational strategies, which is familiar and comfortable territory where a consensus on action is more easily achieved.

I resist those objections and hesitations. My own experience in talking for years with physicians about end-of-life care has persuaded me that many worry at great length about how they should respond to dying patients—with death itself part of the trouble but difficult to fully articulate. I have heard many voice in private just the viewpoint expressed in Iona Heath's article, but which has rarely made it out into the public space of a leading medical journal. I count that as an important breakthrough, but it can seem like the kind of thing that a modern doctor should not say: patients do not ordinarily go to doctors to be told that, however your present treatment goes, something or else will sooner or later get you anyway. Yet her aim is not to spread fatalism, gloom, and doom around, but instead to lead us to a shift in priorities in the name of equality, to concentrate on reducing premature death, "and to resist the inappropriate accusations of ageism."[20] The latter of course is an allusion to the demographic reality that most money is now spent on the care of the elderly with chronic illnesses, exactly the same place we find the highest portion of end-of-life decisions.

Once the door is further opened to that way of thinking, there are many other suppressed or overlooked questions that need to be pursued. To what extent should present research priorities shift from a focus on the chronic diseases because to not only premature death but also because of all those other pathologies that do not kill but badly cripple the mind and body, such as depression, arthritis, Parkinson's disease, and frailty in the elderly? Can we find better ways of projecting the downward slope of critical illness to make possible an earlier start to end-of-life care, even running the risk of stopping life-sustaining too early, not necessarily a worse fate than stopping it too late?

Can we persuade the public that, unless we control the ever-rising costs of care for the chronically ill elderly, and to control the costs of the technological wizardry designed to keep them alive (and giving us in the process ethical and medical fits in managing their end-of-life care), that the entire health care system will be in jeopardy? We can try.

I said early on in this paper that if we open up the problem of death in our lives and health care and the cherished belief that more medical progress is the best way to deal with it, the results could be revolutionary. I do not believe we have a choice. If we do not do so, then end-of-life care will continue to mercilessly vex us, health care costs will rise to prohibitive heights, and our lives will be the worse for it. Less is more.

*References*

1. P. R. Orzag and E. J. Emanuel, "Health Care Reform and Cost Control," *New England Journal of Medicine 373*, no. 7 (2010): 601–603.
2. L. R. Sugarman, S. L. Decker, and A. Bercovitz, "Demographic and Social Characteristics and Spending at the End of Life," *Journal of Pain and Symptom Management* 38, no. 1 (2009): 15–26, at 16.
3. *Id.*
4. Congressional Budget Office, *Technological Change and the Growth of Health Care Spending*, Washington, D.C., 2008, at 13.
5. J. Lynn, "Living Long in Fragile Shape: The New Demographics Shape End of Life Care," in B. Jennings, G. E. Kaebnick, and T. Murray, "Improving End of Life Care: Why Has It Been So Difficult?" *The Hastings Center Report Special Supplement Special Report* 35, no. 6 (2005): S14-S18, at S17.
6. D. Cutler, *Your Money or Your Life: Strong Medicine for America's Health Care System* (New York: Oxford University Press, 2004): at 62.
7. J. P. Newhouse, "Medical Care: How Much Welfare Loss?" *Journal of Economic Perspectives* 6, no. 3 (1992): 3–21.
8. D. Callahan, *Taming the Beloved Beast: How Medical Technology Costs Are Destroying Our Health Care System* (Princeton: Princeton University Press, 2009): at 47.

9. M. Andrews, "Rather Than Creating 'Death Panels,' New Law Adds to End-of-Life Provisions," *Washington Post, September 7,* 2010.

10. M. Kim, R. J. Blendon, and J. M. Berenson, "How Interested Are Americans in New Technologies?" *Health Affairs* 20, no. 5 (2001): 194–201, at 200.

11. *Id.,* at 200.

12. J. K. Shim, A. J. Russ, and S. R. Kaufman, "Risk, Life Extension and the Pursuit of Medical Possibilities," *Sociology of Health and Illness* 28, no. 4 (2006): 475–502, at 490.

13. M. Chernew, "Barriers to Constraining Health Care Cost Growth," *Health Affairs* 23, no. 6 (2004): 122–128, at 123.

14. A. Bennett, "End of Life Warning at $618,616 Makes Me Wonder If It Was Worth It," Bloomberg News, available at <http://www.bloomberg.com/apps/news?pid=newsarchive&sid=avRF GNF6Qw_w> (last visited February 11, 2011).

15. D. Rieff, *Swimming in a Sea of Death* (New York: Simon & Schuter, 2008).

16. K. Butler, "My Father's Broken Heart," *New York Times Magazine,* August 24, 2010.

17. W. Haseltine, quoted in M. Fisher, "The Race to Cash In on the Genetic Code," *New York Times,* August 21, 1991.

18. I. Heath, "What Do We Want to Die From?" *British Medical Journal* 341 (2010): c3883.

19. J. H. Muller and B. Koenig, "On the Boundary of Life and Death: The Definition of Dying by Medical Residents," in M. Lock and D. Gordon, eds., *Biomedicine Reconsidered* (Dordrecht: Kluwer Academic Press, 1998): at 369.

20. See Heath, *supra* note 18.

# 7

# DEATH, MOURNING, AND
# MEDICAL PROGRESS

In his splendid book, *The Hour of Our Death* (1981), the French historian Philippe Aries noted "the persistence of an attitude toward death that remained almost unchanged for thousands of years, an attitude that expressed a naive acceptance of destiny and nature" (p. 1). That attitude, he argued, created what he called the "tame death." It was marked by the individual's and the community's acceptance of his unalterable fate and its domestication in rituals of mourning. Death was given a formal and acknowledged status in the life of human communities.

There was a "familiar simplicity" about death, to use Aries's expression. It was not simply an individual, private loss but was taken as a blow to all those who survived, both family and strangers. Death required a public affirmation of human solidarity against a harsh and indifferent nature. It was not to be hidden: families should be there when death was at hand, and the door thrown open to neighbors and even those passing by in the street.

The "tame death," Aries contended, has in modern countries—but especially in Europe and America—has been replaced by a "wild death," with death to be rejected, evaded, rationalized, and hidden. Aries's book took death up to the 1970s, and it was that era and its emerging attitudes and practices that he was trying to capture with the notion of a "wild death."

## THE TRANSITIONAL DEATH:
## REFORMING THE CARE OF THE DYING

I want to bring that story up to date. We are, I believe, now moving on to another stage, one marked by medicine's de facto rejection at the research level of the ancient belief that death is inevitable, an immutable and unchangeable fact and human fate. It is a stage that simultaneously displays considerable ambivalence about the "hour of our death," about appropriate modes of mourning, and about the place of death in the life of the community. Once again we are being forced to ask some old questions. What is the meaning and significance of death for us as individuals? How might it best be dealt with as a medical challenge? And what does death mean for our public life and cultural practices?

The 1960s and 1970s might well be understood as the transitional era. Death was, to use the cliché of the era, just beginning to come "out of the closet," at least for public discussion. There was a rising tide of complaints about the way people died, often alone in ICUs, wrapped in a harsh cocoon of tubes and wires, their families denied admittance. By that time some 80% of people in the United States were dying in hospitals or nursing homes, and there was no shortage of personal stories of medical indignities, poor palliative care and deficient pain relief, and a chilling indifference to the sensibilities of anxious friends and relatives.

A Pulitzer-prize winning book by psychiatrist Ernest Becker, *The Denial of Death* (1973), well caught the spirit of the times. Out of those complaints came a number of reform efforts: better physician training in the care of the dying, the hospice movement, and a patient rights initiative aiming to give the dying a voice in their final care. But something was missing in most of those efforts. A deep and sustained discussion and consideration of death itself was all but absent. It was still assumed that we would all die, that nothing could be done about that, leaving it up to individuals to make of that reality what they would. The only issue of public interest was how to legally and organizationally traverse the road from life to death.

As that development was taking place, there was a parallel movement as well, a shift in the care of the dead body and in rituals of mourning. In the mid-1940s I witnessed my dead grandmother laid out in an open coffin in her house, her wake open and convenient for all her neighbors. I did not realize that I had seen the final throes of an ancient practice and would never witness that kind of scene again. This being America—with a buck to be made, and many families no longer drawn to dead bodies in the living room—the modern funeral industry arose to tidy up and gloss over death. It did an effective job, embalming and beautifying the corpse, offering elaborate, expensive, and rot-resistant coffins, and a well polished therapeutic professionalism to cope with the mourning self and grieving relatives.

The possibilities for black humor were numerous, and British writers Evelyn Waugh and Jessica Mitford made great fun of it all in their books *The Loved One* (1948) and *The American Way of Death* (1963). More solemnly, Geoffrey Gorer's book *Death, Grief, and Mourning in Contemporary Britain* (1965) described the goal in that country as the banishment of death altogether from the public sphere, aiming to make it invisible. He could have been talking about the United States.

## SHUTTING THE CLOSET DOOR ON DEATH

Mourning started on a parallel track in America. While the funeral industry has continued, large church funerals and graveside rites began to decline in the 1970s, at least with the more educated portion of the population. Private funerals, insistently for families only, increased. Open caskets with visible bodies started going out of fashion, and then—as cremations increased—even closed caskets with intact bodies. There was one final step down that road: a steady rise of memorial services, with no bodies at all. Their aim is less to mourn a death than to celebrate a life. A small minority, even more sophisticated, made clear to one and all that there should be no ceremony of any kind; even a scattering of ashes at sea by a few friends would be going too far. In a word, dear friends, keep your grief to yourselves. The ancient notion of a public death and collective mourning was thus finally turned on its head by these successive developments.

Now I am speaking of trends only, first visible in the 1970s and 1980s, and many traditional wakes and funerals still occur. But the direction seems clear, and what was at first a small trend seems now to have gained momentum. Yet that is not the end of the story, either with death or with mourning. By the 1990s still more changes surfaced, opening up a new chapter on both. The change has at least three important elements: a gradual shift in the palliative care movement, a more aggressive medical and scientific campaign against aging and death, and a growing confusion about mourning.

## THE CHANGING FACE OF PALLIATIVE CARE

The palliative care movement got its initial impetus as a response to a great deal of evidence and anguished, sometimes angry, complaints that pain was often badly managed with the dying and that physicians were poorly trained in relieving pain. A fear of killing patients by excessive use of opioids, and thus some legal threats, did not help matters (though the threats were more fantasy than real). The physician Eric Cassell made an important contribution to the debate with his book *The Nature of Suffering and the Goals of Medicine* (1991) which noted the importance of distinguishing between pain and suffering, too often conflated, by physicians as much as by laypeople.

As the scope of palliative care was broadened by that distinction, it gradually became clear that palliative care was appropriate for all patients, not just with end-of-life care, or only in hospice care. At least in the early reform years, it was understood that a dying patient needed palliative care addressed to both pain and suffering, but also that a key to a good death was its acceptance by patients. As time went on, however, many hospice providers concluded that not all patients can or will accept death, thus breaking with the Aries paradigm of a tame death. Indeed, good palliative care requires careful management of dying patients for whom the inability to accept death is itself a source of suffering.

As palliative care was broadened beyond dying patients, the idea emerged that for some patients—particularly those whose condition is on the borderline between potentially treatable and terminally ill—it would be appropriate to team up a clinician and a palliative care specialist. An analogous problem was identified in hospice care, which had long contended with the fact that too many terminal patients got into hospice much later than would have been ideal, often only during the last week or two of their lives.

An unwillingness to accept the coming of death is usually a prime reason for the delay. Doctors and families are often unable to accept the fact that a patient is dying. But it is also a reflection of the difficulty of discerning a clear borderline between living and dying. In retrospect, it is often possible to say that a patient was over-treated and should have been allowed to die earlier. But it is becoming harder and harder to determine in advance just which patients those are.

## MEDICAL UTOPIANISM: THE WAR AGAINST AGING AND DEATH

The present period might best be characterized as a revolt against death itself, and with that a revolt against the aging that has gradually become death's most common predecessor. Death is gradually being transformed from a fixed and unchangeable biological and human inevitability to a contingent event, even accidental and manipulable. Where death was once thought to be natural and therefore unchangeable, the very notion of "the natural" is vanishing from our vocabulary, or at least from the vocabulary of aggressive medical research.

As William Haseltine, the colorful CEO of Human Genome Sciences, put it a few years ago, "death is nothing but a series of preventable diseases" (Fisher 1999). That statement verges on the ridiculous, but the international biomedical research agenda has targeted every known lethal disease for conquest. With time and adequate financial resources, the belief goes, all of them can be conquered. The leading argument in favor of the $3 billion Human Genome Project, completed a few years ago, was that it would reveal the ultimate genetic source of disease, opening the way for decisive cures. It has not worked out that way—proteins may be more important—but along came stem cell research to stake a new claim of opening the door to a massive saving of lives. That has not quite worked out yet either, but hope springs eternal these days about the potentialities of medical research, as necessary to drive the economic engine of research as it is to sustain critically ill patients.

I will not take up the question of whether such claims are credible, whether in fact death as a biological phenomenon can be eliminated. But hope now has much the same kind of valence in research that medicine has always given it in the care of individual patients. Hope drives good medical care, for the physician and the patient, and now hope also drives the war against aging and disease. The trans-humanism movement, which includes many reputable scientists among its followers, eagerly foresees radically extended life expectancies, the cure of most diseases, and dramatically new power to alter human nature and the human condition. These are not widespread views, nor have they seeped far into the popular consciousness, but they are out there and gaining ground.

None of this might matter but for its spillover effect, or perhaps more precisely because of the way it dovetails with the steady, incremental gains being made in mortality reduction and increasingly long life spans. As a demographic matter, mortality in developed countries is declining because of a combination of improved socioeconomic conditions, disease prevention, behavioral changes, and the provision of organized health care. No end of that progression is in sight. Fewer and fewer demographers believe any longer that there is any fixed limit to average life expectancy, or even with individual life spans. That data has had the effect of encouraging utopian dreams—and who can say that those dreams are totally groundless?

However, I am convinced that the changing research perspective on death has a clinical and cultural corollary, affecting the way death here and now is thought about, or at least tacitly understood. At the practical, clinical level, constant technological innovation has made it increasingly hard to know when someone is dying; the line between living and dying has become steadily more obscure. Why is that? Whatever the lethal, terminal condition, there is almost always something technological that can be done to give the patient a few more days, or weeks, or months. Cancer therapy, with an endless number of experimental treatments, is a fine example. It is easy to persuade patients, their families, and their doctors not to give up hope: let's try it even if the odds are not good—and yet not impossible either. For desperate patients, worried families, and aggressively acculturated oncologists, that is too often an irresistible argument. I paid a last visit to an old friend a few years ago, a pioneer in bioethics who had taught courses for medical students on end-of-life care. He could not speak well, his mouth filled with sores. I asked him why. His doctors were, he said, trying one more round of experimental chemotherapy. "Why did you allow that?" I asked with some astonishment. A bit sheepishly he answered, "Well, they talked me into it." He died a week later.

## THE MEDICAL SCHISM

There is a profound schism now at the very heart of medicine. The palliative care movement has been working its way backwards in history, aiming to return to a tame death. In contrast, what I call the research imperative moves forward in time, implicitly aiming to conquer death one disease at a time. Few researchers will say that is their aim, but the logic of the medical research enterprise pushes it in that direction. Those of us who are skeptical of that venture have been given some names: we are called "mortalists" for accepting death as human given, and "apologists" for defending that awful state of affairs (Overall 2003).

The net result of the schism, pulling medicine in two contradictory directions, cannot fail to express itself at the bedside. One can see the tension at work in our ordinary language, where we commend both the person who dies with quiet resignation and the person who fights death to the end. Which stance are we supposed to take these days when a lethal disease comes upon us? Fight or give up?

In his book *Swimming in a Sea of Death* (2008), writer David Rieff describes the illness and eventual death of his mother, the writer Susan Sontag, from cancer, and her unwavering refusal to accept its inevitability. She lost the struggle but never gave up trying. Her story helps to qualify the widespread—and false—belief that hardly anyone wants an all-out effort to salvage life when death is on its way. In the 1970s, patients complained about doctors who would not let dying people die. Much more common now are the complaints of doctors about patients or their families who want everything possible done to save their lives. In Sontag's case, it was irrelevant to her that the available (and ultimately fruitless) treatments could themselves be a misery, and there may be a growing number of those who feel the same way.

Where does that leave grief and mourning? In a confusing place, I believe. If death is increasingly seen as a biological accident, a contingent and not necessarily fixed part of our human fate, then how are we to mourn those who die? How, that is, are we to come to terms with deaths that might now have been averted, but which also, even if not avoidable now, may well be so in the future? What is the meaning of death in a utopia-driven scientific age?

## HOW WE DIE AND HOW WE MOURN: LET ME COUNT THE WAYS

I want to get at those questions by noting the various ways in which death comes upon us, particularly centering on disease in comparison with other forms of death. Until I began developing some lists, aiming for a kind of typology of death, I had not realized how varied its forms can be, and how equally varied our response to them can be. I will quickly run through my list, which could, with a bit of imagination, be made even longer.

There is *death from disease* (in childhood, adulthood, old age, and from preventable, curable, and unavoidable disease; and there is sudden or foreseeable death from disease); *death from natural disaster* (hurricanes, floods, drought, volcanic eruptions; and avoidable versus unavoidable risks); *death from war and political upheavals* (wars, riots, genocide, and holocausts); *death from criminal violence* (murder, gang wars); *death from suicide* (among the young, adults, the elderly); and *death from accidents* (auto accidents, falls, poisoning, fires, drowning).

Each one of those deaths can bring different kinds of grief and mourning. I give only some examples from my own life:

- the quick death of my 86-year-old mother from colon cancer with little suffering;
- the sudden and wholly unexpected death of my six-week-old son from sudden infant death syndrome (SIDS), a condition still with no known cause or cure;
- the deaths of three young friends and two colleagues from suicide;
- the death of three children of friends from drug overdose in the 1970s;
- the death of two teenage children of friends from auto accidents;
- the deaths of many old friends and acquaintances from cancer and heart disease, the most common diseases of the elderly;
- the death by murder of a college student daughter of a friend;
- the sudden death a day after giving birth of a daughter-in-law from a pulmonary embolism after a C-section.

The severity of grief in each of those cases was different, from mild to severe, and the length and intensity of mourning no less varied. One does not quickly get over the death of children or sudden, unexpected premature deaths. And people vary enormously in their resilience and in the meaning they attach to death.

Which deaths are better and worse? The death of an elderly person from a common disease of aging seems far better accepted than the death of the young by violence. I can hardly imagine what it is like to see one's family and children tortured and then murdered before one's eyes in genocidal killing. Nor have I been able to get out of mind a recent news story about a father who accidentally drove over and killed his eight-year-old daughter playfully hiding in a pile of leaves in a driveway.

### WHAT MIGHT HAVE BEEN: ITS IMPACT ON MOURNING

But there are certain kinds of death that seem to torture people in a way particularly hard to endure. I will call them the "it might have been otherwise" deaths. By that I mean those deaths that might have been prevented, and I want to distinguish two types of such deaths. One of them is no doubt as old as human beings, that of the accidental death that could have been prevented: the parent who did not notice the small child getting too near the water or too near the fireplace, or the driver who took his eyes off the road a moment too long.

The other type has become steadily more common in modern medicine and bears on my notion of death as an accidental, contingent matter, no longer a matter of inescapable fate. I will call it the "it can be otherwise" death. Preventive medicine is now filled with examples. Colon cancer, which killed my mother at a time when there were no early diagnostic procedures, can now be readily detected by sigmoidoscopy or colonoscopy, and if detected early enough, it can be cured in most cases. Changes in unhealthy behavior, such as smoking, a lack of exercise, or a poor diet, can save thousands of lives. Drugs for high blood pressure and cholesterol can avert death from heart disease. The message from modern preventive medicine, in sum, is that if one takes care of oneself, makes use of available disease screening technologies, and uses the right combination of drugs, then death is not so inevitable after all.

The research imperative and the hope invested in it is another manifestation of deaths that could be otherwise. Advocates for stem cell research look to regenerative medicine to save many lives, from heart disease and diabetes to Alzheimer's disease. When our 42-day-old child died from SIDS, my wife and I could do nothing but mourn and go on to have other children. It did not cross our minds 40 years ago to lobby the National Institutes of Health to create a research program to find a cure; for us, it was just something terrible that could happen to new babies, to be endured and accepted.

More recently, however, my wife was recruited by a much younger woman who had just lost a child from SIDS. She wanted help in raising research money for a cure, creating a small private foundation for that purpose. I don't know how common it is in other countries, but it is striking now how many people in the United States who lose family members join advocacy groups to raise research money. The advocacy drive for stem cell research has been heavily financed by patient advocacy groups, intent on finding cures for lethal disease. Many obituaries now regularly carry a request that I believe was entirely absent when I was growing up: please make contributions to the American Heart Association or the American Cancer Society or some other disease-oriented advocacy group.

One advocacy group for stem cell research has talked of the possibility of saving 130 million American lives if it is successful. Such optimism is hyperbolic, but there is much of it about. Disease ought not to be accepted, resignation is no longer acceptable—and fate is now in human hands. That is the new spirit.

## WRESTLING WITH FATE

The perceptive political scientist Michael Walzer (1983) has well caught the essence of this new spirit. "What has happened in the modern world," he writes, "is that disease itself, even when it is endemic rather than epidemic, has come to be seen as a plague. And since the plague can be dealt with, it must be dealt with. People will no longer endure what they no longer believe they have to endure" (p. 8).

Yet think a moment about the new configuration of death and its implications for grief and mourning. People have long believed, even against the depressing history of mankind, that war and the deaths they cause *need* not happen. Peace is possible, and in some places in the world it actually exists. Death from social violence is no less avoidable: some countries have a vanishingly low murder and violence rate. Good mental health programs can reduce the incidence of suicide.

Again and again the message is, death need not be. Even natural disasters are not wholly beyond human reach. If there is not much that can be done to stop hurricanes or tornadoes, droughts, or floods, sturdier buildings and similar measures can reduce the death rate and, in any case, people can move away from the most hazardous areas. If droughts cannot be stopped, humanitarian social policies can considerably reduce their deadly impact. What about accidents? Even there much advice is available on avoiding auto accidents, falls on slippery floors, and the hazards of leaving windows open when little children are about. So far as I can make out, accidents are an inescapable part of life, but that is rarely said in the literature and homilies on their avoidance—wholly possible, the safety literature implies.

Disease and the decline of the human body have almost become the last frontier of avoidable death. The premise of a tame death was that death simply is part of life, to be lived and died with—and to be suitably mourned along with the many other ways death can come to us. Now that frontier is being breached. There is no disease that is thought to be in principle incurable, no form of biological death that is not taken to be conquerable.

The "what might have been" of careful preventive foresight to avert death and the "what might be" of promising research have come together, leaving us in a new land. It is not quite a land where death is no more, and no doubt never will be, but it is one where the main ingredients of a peaceful death, acceptance and resignation, have been declared socially toxic and individually passé. We "mortalists" and "apologists" are, so to speak, ought to be a dying breed.

## MOURNING IN A NEW LAND

Where does that leave grief and mourning? It is surely harder, I think, to devise rituals of mourning in a world where less and less can be attributed to fate and chance, and where the scope of human causality, responsibility, and culpability grows ever larger.

The distinctive feature of the death of my mother at 86 was that it was treated as a natural event. Sadness was in order: she was loved and would be missed, but there were no tears, no obvious grief. Life is meant to go on. But that viewpoint will not be easy to sustain in a world of ever-improving diagnostic and screening possibilities: deaths like hers need not happen in the future.

There will be more space for regret about what might have been avoided, and more space for a mourning marked by anger that an avertable accident had happened. More space for the families of Alzheimer's patients to rage against inadequate research budgets, and more space for the families of those dying from congestive heart failure to resent the failure of cardiologists, however hard they tried, to keep their loved ones alive. But the test is not how hard one tries—only success counts. As Michael Ignatieff (1988) has acutely put it, "the modern world, for very good reasons, does not have a vernacular of fate. Cultures that live by the values of self-realization and self-mastery are not very good at dying, at submitting to those experiences where freedom ends and biological fate begins... their weak side is submitting to the inevitable."

If that is so, and if death itself is being removed from the realm of fate, then what are we supposed to do? We can simply reject the notion that the mastery of fate—if defined as full control of our lives, social and biological—is nearly at hand, or that it ever will be. We might agree that medical progress is an open, endless frontier while at the same time recognizing that death will still come whatever we do. It is thus no less certain that we will need rituals of mourning. Grief will never be cured by science.

Life improved greatly in the 20th century, from increased life expectancy to advances in almost every category of life: housing, recreation, income, education, scientific knowledge, and so on. Not only in the developed countries, but increasingly in most developing countries as well, life continues to get better. When I once asked my mother, born in 1895, whether life had improved since her childhood, it took her only a fraction of second to answer decisively: yes. But optimism about the human condition in light of those improvements needs a dose of reality: along with an overall improvement in quality of life, the 20th century witnessed the largest and worst world wars in history, as well as impressive scientific gains in the capacity to kill people in large numbers by use of the most advanced scientific knowledge, whether in physics, which gave us nuclear weapons, or biology, which has given us new tools for biological warfare. People, I have noticed, continue to die—later to be sure, but they are finally and irrevocably dead nonetheless—from all those preventable accidents and diseases and from all of those potentially curable diseases, many of them, like AIDS, subject to the genius of constantly mutating viruses.

I live in an apartment full of elderly people, of which I am one. The disabilities of aging have been pushed back a few years, and high-technology medicine can get my neighbors through many episodes of a kind that killed their parents. But there they are by their 80s (and often earlier): no longer on the tennis courts, using canes and walkers, taking many drugs, enduring some kind of pain or disability (no one suffers from nothing at all), fearful when the elevators are not working that they may have to use the stairs, and of course many of them are already showing early symptoms of dementia. While the New York marathon seems to feature at least one person over 90 each year, those in our apartment house at that age rarely make it out of their apartments, and their dementia is more advanced. Whether that kind of life should be counted a medical triumph remains an open question.

## DEATH: LATER RATHER THAN SOONER, BUT NOT ABOLISHED

The fact that biological fate now comes later, with perhaps some of its harsh edges softened, is not the same as overcoming that fate. We cannot live here and now on promises for the future, all those diseases that will someday be cured. The trouble with nature, the source of our fate, is that it is ingenious in its gifts and its hazards.

That nature beyond our own gives us storms and droughts and disease, show-ing us that it can kill us just as effectively as the most well-organized genocide. As the surprising, unforeseen advent of AIDS made perfectly clear, nature is capa-ble of throwing us curve balls. It has destroyed the reigning myth of the 1960s that infectious disease was all but conquered, and that the remaining chronic and degenerative pathologies of aging would be banished no less quickly. It turns out that as many people may now die of infectious disease as 40 years ago, helped along by AIDS, other new infectious conditions, hospital pathogens, and antibi-otic resistance.

My modest conclusion about the present state of the human condition is that nothing will do away with death and the need for mourning. I use the word need to suggest three thoughts: we are better off if we do not try to explain away death itself as an accident; better off as individuals if we mourn the death of others; and better off when our mourning is public and nourished. Death is still a zero-sum game. To be cured of one disease is to be set up for death by another. To have our life saved from an accident or an earthquake, war or murder, is to increase the odds that we will then die from disease. "He can run but he can't hide," the boxer Joe Louis once said of an opponent before a fight, and that can be said of efforts to save lives as well.

It is surely better to have a longer rather than a shorter life, to die from cancer rather than murder, pneumonia rather than genocide, and to suffer from less pain rather than more. But all that just tinkers with and modifies our fate. Our fate is still death.


## IN PRAISE OF MOURNING

If what I say is true, then it is important that we learn how to restore mourn-ing to its rightful and sensible place, making death tame once again. The old-fashioned way makes more sense than the modern way. An open casket reminds us that the dead person was an embodied person. A funeral service, religious or secular, is better than a later memorial service. Time distances us from those who have died, softening our sense of loss and the sharpness of our grief. That grief fades is of course a blessing in the long run; enduring grief can be destructive. All the more reason then to catch it with a funeral when it is still sharply etched.

Our obituaries should be interesting and readable, as is the case with those in the better British press. Our deaths should bring us to life for those who did not know us. If we die in old age of some disease that most commonly afflicts the elderly, we should ask that contributions be made to groups and organizations helping the young. Flowers should still be acceptable. If we made it to old age, we had our goodly share of life. We should help the young to be so lucky.

Can we restore death as a public event? Not easily, but a few steps in that direction might help. We could begin by asking that no one should ask us to ignore his death, insisting that there be no funeral or memorial service. It seems to me an insult to one's own self-worth and self-respect to deny family and friends the privilege and comfort of grieving together, to ask in effect to be instantly forgotten—a strange kind of self-destructive narcissism.

At the least, we should recognize that once we have died, our problems and feelings have come to an end. That is rarely true with the survivors, and minimal decency seems to me to require that their needs be recognized. The famous Washington hostess, Alice Roosevelt Longworth, daughter of Theodore Roosevelt, left instructions that at her death there was to be no funeral, no ceremonies of any kind, and she got her way. A friend, however, felt that was wrong: "I think it was a great mistake...it was hard on everybody....Maybe she did not want people to say pompous things about her. But I think when someone is not given a farewell you have a terribly uneasy feeling of their spirit hovering. It is as if a piece of music stopped before the final chord" (Felsenthal 1988, p. 268).

We could also usefully restore the practice of hanging black crepe on the door of the home of the deceased, announcing to all of one's neighbors that a death has occurred and that family and friends are in mourning. While an Irish custom I heard about as a child probably went too far—that of a wake featuring the deceased propped up in a chair at the center of the event—the idea had a certain mischievous charm. Beyond those ideas a final suggestion: keep those public funerals and open coffins. Then hold a party on the anniversary of a person's death. Just have a good time in his or her honor. It will be more fun than most memorial services, and serious, shared grief will have been well served earlier.

## References

Aries, P. 1981. *The hour of our death,* trans. Helen Weaver. New York: Knopf, p. 1.

Becker, E. 1973. *The denial of death.* New York: Free Press.

Cassell, E. 1991. *The nature of suffering and the goals of medicine.* New York: Oxford Univ. Press.

Felsenthal, C. 1988. *Alice Roosevelt Longworth.* New York: Putnam.

Fisher, L. 1999. The place to cash in on the genetic code. *NY Times,* Aug. 29.

Gorer, G. 1965. *Death, grief, and mourning in contemporary Britain.* London: Cresset Press.

Ignatieff, M. 1988. Modern dying. *New Republic,* Dec. 26.

Mitford, J. 1963. *The American way of death.* New York: Simon & Schuster.

Overall, C. 2003. *Aging, death and human longevity.* Berkeley: Univ. of California Press.

Rieff, D. 2008. *Swimming in a sea of death.* New York: Simon & Schuster.

Walzer, M. 1983. *Spheres of justice: A defense of pluralism and equity.* New York: Basic Books.

Waugh, E. 1948. *The loved one: An Anglo-American tragedy.* Boston: Little Brown.

# 8

## TERMINATING LIFE-SUSTAINING TREATMENT OF THE DEMENTED

Some subjects in ethics elicit a far greater degree of emotional discomfort than others. It is not the delicacy or complexity of the subject as such that seems to be the problem. It is, instead, a tacit recognition that, try as we might, it is especially hard to disentangle our personal response from the issues themselves. And this makes it especially hard to avoid self-deception and self-interest in our analysis.

Terminating life-sustaining treatment for demented patients is such an issue. Dementia is universally feared, more so than almost any other disease. Few of us can tolerate the thought that we might become its victim. Even if we can bring love and devotion to the care of those with dementia, they can in turn elicit in us the fear that we might someday be ourselves so afflicted, and they can incite a sense of loathing and horror, usually despite ourselves. We cannot easily distinguish our own feelings about the condition from what is the actual good of the patient. The harder it is for us to imagine life as tolerable in such circumstances, the harder it will be to determine what is beneficial for the patient.

This same troubling dimension will, analogously, almost surely begin playing itself out in the years to come on the social and economic level, as a combination of increased numbers and likely higher costs for the care of those afflicted with dementia becomes a more explicit agenda item for resource allocation. Will society show the same kind of ambivalence, self-questioning, and anguish felt by many individuals as it further develops policies and spending patterns? If so, how will it incline in its values and predilections, with increased generosity or discreet withdrawal?

The general question I want to pursue is this: under what circumstances should life-sustaining treatment for dementia patients be ended and the patients allowed to die? The more specific, troubling, question is: ought the fact of dementia make a difference in our decision, distinguishing it from other termination situations? These questions would have been much easier to deal with ten or fifteen years ago. They are harder now for three reasons—reasons which, vexingly enough, move in different, conflicting directions. The first reason is that recent research on Alzheimer disease is beginning to show that much more can be done for its sufferers than was previously possible and that a viable, even if crippled, self may endure far later into the disease process than was earlier believed. The second reason is that new sensibilities about disabled populations have emerged over the past few decades that have alerted us to the possibility of stigmatizing and demeaning the demented, thus worsening their situation. The third reason is that, one way or another, health care resources will become more limited in the future, and the explicit, open rationing of health care more certain; dementia is not likely, nor should it be spared from scrutiny in that process. It would be ideal to develop a way of thinking about Alzheimer that managed to take on all three of these problems simultaneously despite their potential conflict, seeing if they can be dealt with in a way that is integrated and coherent.

I will initially sketch a context to help situate the care of dementia patients and the termination of their treatment. Then I will move on to develop some criteria to make termination decisions.

## A CONTEXT FOR ANALYSIS

The pertinent context here is three fold: (1) our knowledge of the inner life, and selfhood, of those suffering from dementia (by which I will primarily mean Alzheimer disease); (2) the messages, symbolic and literal, about dementia that could be conveyed to society by alternative kinds of policies and practices; and (3) the economic considerations involved in making decisions about the good of individual patients.

*Dementia and the Self.* Two major problems need to be noted. One of them, to which I will not devote much attention, bears on the place and force of advance directives in the care of the demented. Ideally, people should draw up advance directives, either a living will or the appointment of a surrogate to act in their behalf should they become incompetent. Those advance directives should stipulate what one wants done in the case of dementia (and I will take it for granted that most, but not all people are not likely to want aggressive life-saving or life-extending treatment with advanced dementia).

Yet there is a potential puzzle here, nicely brought out in the writings of Ronald Dworkin and Sanford H. Kadish, both distinguished legal scholars. At issue is whether the patient's earlier advance directive or the patient's presently expressed or implied desires (assuming the latter differ from the former) should be the determining consideration in decisions to terminate treatment. This situation presents no dilemma if the patient cannot express desires at all, but does if the patient states a desire to continue living, or if behavioral evidence suggests that the patient is satisfied enough with his present condition and seems to have no urge to be dead.

Dworkin distinguishes between a patient's "experiential" interests—the patient's present state of experienced pleasure, pain, or satisfaction—and the patient's "critical" interests—those interests expressive of a patient's long-standing, settled convictions about what he values in life.[1] An advance directive signed while a patient was in good health and that reflects some carefully thought out personal values could come into conflict with the actual condition and inclinations of a patient at a critical moment. If I have stated while in good health, and after careful reflection, that I would not care to have my life extended if I become demented, should that declaration be respected even if, when the time comes, I seem to be happy enough in my demented state? Dworkin takes the position that the critical interests should be determinative, representing the settled convictions of a patient, and thus that the advance directive should be respected.

Kadish takes the other side, and I believe has the better argument.[2] His reasons bear on the selfhood of the demented person—a self he presumes continues to exist, even if incompetent. It is perfectly possible that we may now find acceptable a life we had earlier judged to be unacceptable, and that we could not have known in advance that such a change in our judgment was possible. As such, it would seem unduly rigid, even doctrinaire, to deny evidence of a dementia patient doing better than he could have anticipated. But what if a patient had foreseen exactly this kind of a possibility and still wanted termination? Doesn't the "critical interest" position encompass just this possibility? Even so, we are still left with a problem: how can someone in any rational way irrevocably determine well in advance what they will want in a situation they have never experienced before? We would do well to be suspicious of such earlier declarations when the evidence before our eyes is that of a patient doing reasonably well and not obviously seeking death. A second reason for resisting Dworkin's position is that a key feature in the development of advance directives has been to stress the possibility of changing or revoking those directives at any time while capacitated, not to assume that they are to function in a fixed, unchangeable way. That same reasoning could be extended to include behavior of the incapacitated that would imply either a change of mind or an implicit unwillingness to see the original criteria of the advance directives invoked in actuality. But I will not explore the problem of advance directives any further here other than to note that how we analyze the problem will, in great part, turn on our interpretation of the selfhood of demented patients, and what various states of that selfhood might morally entail.

I will instead focus my analysis on what should be done when we have no prior knowledge of a person's wishes about termination or even about the person's values. I am thus taking on a hard but not uncommon kind of case, where it is left entirely to us to decide what to do based on our own values or, more precisely, on those values we conscientiously believe should apply in these cases. This focus also helps to bring in sharp relief how we might best think about dementia and termination of treatment. The tendency in much of the discussion of termination is to focus on patient wishes, known or inferred. Obviously that is important but, in the long run, what patients and would-be patients decide is in their best interests, or their ideas of the kind of life best worth living, will be a function of how we come to think of a life weighted down with dementia. What *ought* I to want when I am dying of dementia? That question will also hover just below the surface. We cannot achieve a perfect dissociation of our judgment about ourselves and our judgment about other people; and it would be insensitive to accept a perfect bifurcation.

I begin with my first background question: How are we best to understand the selfhood of the demented person and understand it at different stages in the development of dementia? In what sense can it be said that the demented person has a self? I will here define full selfhood as the capacity to have feelings and to be aware of them, to reason and be able to make decisions, and to enter into relationships with other persons. A person who has even one of those capacities can be said to have a self, even if limited and impaired.

The moral corollary of this definition of selfhood is that, unlike the person in a persistent vegetative state, a person with even a minimal self should be assumed to have the same desire to live as those of us more fortunate to have a full self. We have no reason to think otherwise. There should be, that is, the same presumption in favor of treatment as would be the case with anyone else. I stress "presumption" here to indicate that there can be reasons to overturn that presumption, including inferred evidence from the emotional or other expressions of the patient himself, a point to which I will return later.

What can be said of the selfhood of those suffering dementia? Recent scientific evidence and more careful patient analysis is beginning to show that the reality may be more complex, less wholly destructive, and more open to intervention than was previously believed, especially if strong efforts are made to work therapeutically with the patient. Joseph Foley strikes a note of caution about the conventional pessimism in this respect. "We too often assume," he writes, "that the absence of emotional display means that no emotion is being experienced. We too often assume that because communication is absent, internal mental process has stopped."[3] Foley does not claim that we know what is going on inside the mind of the demented person. He stresses instead two important points. The first is the lack of good research on the insight of the demented person into his own condition. This deficit in our knowledge is striking when compared with the emphasis on self-understanding found, for example, in psychiatry or psychology more generally. The second is the importance of recognizing the variability, from patient to patient and time to time, in the dementia of the individual patient. No less significant, "it is important to identify functions that are lost, but even more so to identify functions that are preserved." Rebecca Dresser, in her masterful explanation of the possibility of insight into the mind of demented persons, concludes that "we can achieve adequate evidentiary ground for judgments on the nature of life from the patient's point of view."[4]

Tom Kitwood and Kathleen Bredin, of the Bradford Dementia Group at Bradford University in England, strike an even more optimistic note. They emphasize a number of points: that there can be a considerable reversal of even severely deteriorated patients when their social relationships and conditions of life are changed; that the condition can be stabilized in those given an intensive program of activities; and that some animal studies show the significant positive effect of companionship and activity and an improved environment.[5] They conclude that "Evidence from the care context, then, is beginning to suggest that a dementing illness is not necessarily a process of inevitable and global deterioration."

In still another study, Steven R. Sabat and Rom Harré provide evidence to show that the self of personal identity "persists far into the end stage of the disease." The self, they contend, can be lost, "but only indirectly as a result of the disease. The primary cause of the loss of self is the ways in which others view and treat the Alzheimer sufferer."[6] Victoria Cotrell and Richard Schulz add still another dimension, focusing on the active role of patients in shaping a response to their condition. "The inherent message," they write, "is that individuals with dementia are important actors responding and adapting to the disease, rather than passive individuals who are succumbing to deficits."[7] Taken together, these two perspectives have the potential to transform common attitudes toward those with dementia. How we as family and friends and caretakers think about and respond to the demented patient will make a difference in the self-perception of the patient, and that self-perception is itself potentially amenable to alteration by the patient herself.

The evidence cited in these articles is not definitive, and the authors do not make such a claim. But it is surely sufficient to suggest that, for ethical purposes, the sufferer of dementia cannot decisively be declared either out of touch with himself or definitively out of the human community (especially since communication, however rudimentary, with dementia patients remains possible almost to the very end). As outside observers, we may be appalled by the kind of self we observe, even fearful; but this is *our* reaction, not necessarily that of the demented person to herself. A distinction must of course be made between the earlier and later stages of the condition, and it is surely possible that by the last stages the deterioration is so far advanced that the familiar stereotype is realized: that of a person whose deterioration has destroyed both her body and her self. Even then we may not know exactly when the self was irretrievably lost, when some significant borderline was crossed.

I draw from this analysis one simple conclusion: There is no self-evident reason why, based on the selfhood of the dementia victim, he or she should be treated in any significantly different way from any other incapacitated patient. In early stages of the disease, there is less and less reason now to write off the patient as beyond useful therapy or to excuse caretakers from making vigorous efforts to promote the most supportive environment for the patient. Even as the disease progresses, the possibility of useful intervention remains. Only when the patient is in the late stages of the disease, wholly out of contact with those around him, is it legitimate to change course; and then comfort care only is appropriate. Even at the latest stage, however, the demented patient should clearly be distinguished from the (carefully diagnosed) persistent vegetative state patient, when all possibility of selfhood has almost certainly been lost. It is doubtful there could ever be a comparable level of certainty with dementia patients.

This conclusion presupposes a partial answer to a question posed at the outset, whether the fact of dementia, as distinguished from other medical conditions, should make a difference in our decisions to terminate treatment. If the most important issue is the selfhood of a patient, then dementia poses problems no different in kind from those posed by other medical conditions or situations where the disease is degenerative, the future bleak, and the patient increasingly incompetent. We can well understand the special fear that we all have about becoming demented and the profound assault of dementia upon the integrity of the self. Yet I find it hard to identify a feature of dementia that makes it singularly different from other diseases that can bring about a destruction of the mind and then the body such that some special standards are needed.

At the same time, however, something about the constellation of symptoms and losses seems to make the whole of the illness greater than the sum of the parts; therein may lie its special horror. That horror, nonetheless, is not sufficient to justify some idiosyncratic dementia standards for termination of treatment. On the contrary, because of the fear and dread the disease inspires, every effort should be made to work against these fears and to treat the dementia patient similarly to other patients.

*Public Meaning and Public Symbols.* In the case of dementia, we face an old public dilemma. There is an ancient theological saying that we should love the sinner but not the sin. Paraphrased for my purposes, our public dilemma is this: how are we to work against dementia as a disease while not at the same time coming to slight or demean those who suffer from it or to create excessive anxiety on the part of those who might one day come down with it? A fear of dementia already seems to be a potent force behind the desire of many to legalize euthanasia and physician-assisted suicide. A death in the throes of Alzheimer disease is seen as the mark of a "death without dignity" with first the self destroyed and then the body, leaving only a wreck of a person to go to his death.

The policies we come to adopt about the termination of treatment of the demented will come to play both a literal role in the way we care for them and a symbolic role in indicating how we have come to situate and value them. The symbolism could develop in three possible directions.

First, if we make it much easier to terminate treatment of the demented than other classes of incompetent patients, we will be underscoring our social loathing of the condition and our consequent devaluing of a life burdened with that condition. We will also, on the other side of the ledger, be signaling our desire to reduce the anxiety of those in the earlier stages of the condition, as well as that of family members, about their last days (or months). We will be saying that *this* condition deserves special relief. The dilemma is that the price of reducing the anxiety about having dementia is paid by stigmatizing the condition all the more—and thus possibly, very possibly, making it more difficult to engender the attitudes of social acceptance necessary to make the life of the demented (and their families, who will share in the stigmatization) more tolerable and to attract adequate social resources.

Second, if we treat dementia just like other conditions, giving the benefit of any doubt to the continuation of standard medical treatment, then we will inevitably provoke a continuing (and possibly escalating) terror as the number of demented patients increases with the rise in the proportion of the elderly. More and more of us will see ourselves at risk, particularly if we have been healthy enough to stay alive into our eighties. The source of the terror will be obvious enough: there will be no ready or quick release from the dementia, and the body will be treated as if the self of which it is a part is to be preserved at all costs.

To follow the latter course would be to accept the notion that a self remains almost to the end. And how could we not treat that self, even though diminished,

much like other selves? The dilemma here is clear enough: the price of recognizing an ongoing self may be to (a) undergird the usual forces of technological
medicine, which work with the simple rule "when in doubt, treat," while (b) at
the same time enhancing the fear of the condition by seeming to close off a fast
release from it.

Third, we could develop some kind of compromise position, aiming to mini-
mize further stigmatization of dementia while simultaneously reducing the widespread fear that the life of the demented will be unconscionably prolonged. That
will not be easy to do, but I will propose an approach below that may strengthen
the possibilities in that direction.

**Economics: Priorities and Standards.** There can be little doubt that the United
States, like all other developed countries, faces increasingly heavy economic
pressures on its health care system. The growing number of elderly, particularly
those over age eighty, and the growing number of demented patients as a direct
result of that demographic change, must force some unpleasant choices about the
future care of this population. Increasingly, it is possible to hear people say that,
given a shortage of resources, it makes no sense to invest in extended care for
demented patients, who are a burden upon themselves, their families, and society.
Alternatively, some would say that demented patients should be treated like all
other patients and that, in any case, no price can be put on a human life, damaged
or not If the former view is too crude and insensitive, the latter is increasingly
unrealistic and potentially unjust to other sick people who may be deprived of
needed resources due to an imbalance of care given to the demented.[8] How can
we try to think about this problem?

We can begin by not looking at dementia independently of other grave medical conditions. It is no longer reasonable to consider the economic dimensions of
medical conditions and diseases one at a time, in isolation from each other. That
is, to ask how much money we should spend on dementia apart from all other
medical conditions will get us nowhere (any more than we can say how much
should be spent on cancer apart from any other disease). A health care system
must respond to the aggregate ensemble of conditions, and it must do so by putting them next to each other so that their claims can be seen in a comparative way.
The economists are right with their concept of an opportunity cost, which reflects
an evaluation of how any amount of money spent on one medical condition might
more usefully or fairly (or both) be spent on some other medical condition.

The hard problem is to find a way to implement that insight, in this case to
decide what counts as a reasonable expenditure on the demented population in
comparison with spending comparable funds on other patient populations. Here
again we encounter another problem about assigning a unique status to dementia. Is it so uniquely oppressive and fearful that we should therefore spend more

money on those in its last stages than on other fatal conditions, perhaps simply to avoid the appearance of an invidious comparison between the worth of this life and some other life? Or is its downward course so inevitable and destructive that we should therefore spend less life-prolonging money on it, spending our money where it could do more good? Given the impact on families, I would be inclined toward the latter course, but I cannot find anything specific to dementia that would support this bias, though the burden on the family, an extrinsic but hardly irrelevant consideration, provides a nudge in that direction.

A priority-setting approach, of the kind used in the state of Oregon with its Medicaid program, appears as the most feasible way of managing this problem. How can we rank the different medical conditions, physical and psychological, that afflict people? Which are comparatively more or less important? Such a ranking would encompass public opinion, some form of cost-benefit analysis, the likelihood of efficacious treatment, the degree of pain and suffering a condition brings about, and the like. This is not the place to develop a full theory of priority-setting. My own guess is that public opinion would give a high priority to providing decent nursing and palliative care for demented patients but a much lower priority to the use of expensive medicine to prolong life.

I would argue, in any case, that the expenditure of large amounts of money deliberately to prolong the life of the late-stage demented person would not pass an opportunity cost test or qualify as a high priority matter. The inevitable downhill course of the disease would be one reason: death could not be averted, only delayed; and neither cure of the dementia nor amelioration of its effect could be achieved by deliberate efforts to prolong life. The increasingly diminished selfhood of the patient would be another reason: the more diminished the self, as part of a trajectory of gradual diminishment, the less likely that prolongation would be able even significantly to maintain, much less restore, the selfhood that had been lost. On the contrary, it would seem a perfect example of prolonging an irreversible death. I conclude that society would, under any comparative analysis, most likely conclude that expensive life-extending care for the severely demented—as for any late-stage terminally ill patient—could not compete well in the face of other medical needs. Nor should it. I add here one caveat: to the extent that further research can find ways to improve the life of those with early-stage dementia the claim to resources to do just that would be strong.


## DEVISING CRITERIA FOR TREATMENT TERMINATION

In proposing three contextual and background considerations, I have tried to elaborate on those aspects of dementia that should most concern us in thinking about termination of life-sustaining treatment. The welfare of the demented person must, however, take precedence over other considerations (though not wholly to override them), and thus the question of selfhood is central. But since economic forces will impinge on treatment decisions, and since any policy affecting the demented will telegraph social meanings and symbols, they cannot go unconsidered.

I want now to focus on individual treatment decisions, indicating along the way where the economic and social dimensions might make a difference in the analysis. I will assume that individuals differ in their response to dementia, and that any criteria must have sufficient flexibility to take that into account. I will also assume that the degree to which the disease has advanced will be an important variable; late-stage dementia is not the same as early-stage dementia and that difference counts. I will assume, finally, that whoever is making the termination decision will have done everything possible to take into account the bias of his or her own emotional responses to the patient's condition, recognizing that it is the good of the patient, not that of the decision maker, that matters.

Just because of the problem of bias, it would be unwise to use the notion of "quality of life," commonly used in this kind of a context. Since we do not have good insight into the mind of the demented person, we cannot assume a priori that dementia is inevitably and necessarily experienced by the person himself as a poor quality of life. That may be the case early on with the condition but, ironically, perhaps not so much when the disease is far advanced and the patient is perhaps less aware of his own deterioration. As mentioned above, our lack of insight into the consciousness of the demented person should make us hesitate about quality-of-life judgments. Here in particular lies the temptation to mistake our own distress for and recoil from the patient's condition for that of the patient; the patient may or may not feel the same, and we will have no definitive way of knowing. To the extent that we learn better how to gain such insight, the possibility for a firmer judgment will increase.

Three standards can be proposed for making decisions to terminate treatment: (1) no one should, in the modern world, have to live longer in the advanced stages of dementia than he would have in a pre-technological era; (2) the more advanced the damage of the dementia, the more legitimate it is to overturn the usual bias in favor of treatment; and (3) whoever is making the decision has as strong an obligation to prevent a painful and degrading death as to promote health and life. I will discuss each standard in turn.

**No one should now have to live longer in the advanced stages of dementia turn he would have in a pretechnological era.** Every person suffering from dementia should be given adequate care, comfort, and palliation. That standard should never be changed and always be honored. It has been an enduring goal of medical practice for 2,500 years in the Western world and is particularly pertinent here given the chronic, degenerative nature of the condition. But what about the use of those medical skills and technologies that are the mark of modern medicine and that are ordinarily used to cure disease and to extend life? Are they equally required? They range from the inexpensive, painless use of antibiotics to the more elaborate and expensive techniques of open-heart surgery, dialysis, and organ transplantation.

There can be no obligation, in the later stages of dementia, to prolong with technology—even simple, non-burdensome technologies—the life of someone whose course is most likely going to be steadily downhill, steadily worse. If at all possible, a patient should be spared that likelihood, and thus opportunistic infections, organ failures, and other life threatening conditions should not be opposed with technology (whose use should be restricted to palliation). It is hard to imagine how the use of modern technologies that extend life could be more beneficial for the advanced-stage patient, since such use actually enhances the likelihood of an even worse outcome than its omission. Modern medicine should be an option for severely deteriorated patients only if it promises clear benefit; it should not be an imposed burden. Moreover, the costs of high-technology terminal care are not a trivial consideration. Such costs can be justified only if some clear benefit is to result; and there seems to be none here.

**The likely deterioration in a late-stage demented patient should lead to a shift in the usual standard of treatment, that of stopping rather than continuing treatment.** The ordinary standard of treatment with an incompetent patient is, lacking specific instructions otherwise, to treat rather than not to treat, with the burden of proof on those who would want to stop the treatment. With advanced dementia—as with any irreversible terminal illness in its later stages—that burden should be reversed; that is, the presumption should be against aggressive treatment unless there are some compelling reasons to continue the treatment. The traditional reasoning behind the older and ordinary rule is that most people prefer to go on living rather than dying; thus, it is a not-surprising standard. In this case, where the effect of continuing treatment would be simultaneously to prolong the life and the deterioration of the patient, there can be no obvious benefits. The treatment paves the way for further deterioration, not improvement or even stability. That would seem to be a strange way of honoring the remaining selfhood of the patient, if selfhood there is.

Should, however, there be some degree of reasonable uncertainty about the prognosis of the patient, then there is a middle-way option between aggressive treatment and none at all. In her illuminating and enormously sensible recent book, *Choosing Medical Care in Old Age*, Dr. Muriel Gillick develops the option of "intermediate level care," by which she means conservative, low-technology treatment, and often at home rather than in a hospital. This gives the patient a chance for improvement if the basic biological resiliency is there, but at the same time does not invasively and artificially try to increase the low odds. "We need," she writes, "to accept that a *chance* of recovery is not a sufficient reason to embark on a treatment course if the chance is small, the hazards great, and the patient irreversibly demented."[9] Intermediate-level care provides a prudent way of dealing with those ambiguous situations in which the chance may not be too low. The value of this approach has been partially confirmed in a study comparing outcomes in Dementia Special Care Units, which concentrate on patient comfort, with those in traditional long-term care facilities, which are more open to interventions. The former units, the study found, resulted in both a lower level of patient discomfort and lower costs as well (though there was a higher mortality rate, as might be expected).[10]

**There is as great an obligation to prevent a lingering painful, or degrading death as there is to promote health and life.** Among the important goals of medicine are those of preserving life, sustaining health, and relieving pain and suffering. I propose one other goal: the duty to seek, within moral means, a decent, peaceful death, which is an aspect of the duty to try to relieve suffering. A death that is lingering, painful, or psychologically degrading is not a good death. If medicine fails to do what it can within moral limits to avoid such a death, it has failed in an important part of its mission. This means avoiding a technological obsessiveness that would seek to maintain the body and its organs well past the point of any benefit. It also means encouraging efforts to understand how the continuation of treatment may affect the quality of the death it might make possible or likely.

In thinking about the likely downhill course of the disease, ought the diminished self of the patient make a difference? I am ambivalent on this point. I argued above that, since the demented person has a residual, though severely impaired self, he should be treated like any other impaired person, and treatment continued. But there is a side of me, and of most others I would surmise, that wants to say that the degree of impairment of the self should somehow make a difference in our reckoning. This impulse no doubt springs from a common reaction to the deteriorated self of the demented person: I do not want to end my life like that. Though understandable as an impulse, I can find no good reason to allow it to overcome the previously stated principle that, if there is any self at all, the demented person should not be singled out on the basis of special criteria related to her dementia.

No physician can guarantee a peaceful death, but many things can be done to increase its possibility. The most important is simply to promote a responsibility to balance the possible benefits of continued treatment with the possible harms of worsening the process of dying. Those two possibilities should be set in fruitful tension with each other. This will require asking not simply about the immediate benefit that treatment will bring (for it might reduce a fever or thwart a spreading infection), but also about the long-term consequences of the intervention. A treatment that provides an immediate benefit only to set the patient up for a worse death in the future should not be considered a value for the patient. Nor, economically, can it be considered a desirable social value.

## APPLICATION OF THE CRITERIA

What I am looking for with these criteria is to address three major problems of decisions to terminate treatment: how and when to use available technologies that could sustain the life of the patient; how and when to turn upside down the traditional standard that when in doubt treatment should be provided; and how to determine when to invoke the duty of the physician to help the patient avoid a poor death. At present, treatment is often initiated or sustained because of a pervasive belief that potentially effective treatment should be used, that doubt should be resolved in favor of treatment, and that the physician's primary duty lies in improving or maintaining a decent quality of life rather than in promoting a peaceful death. I do not claim that this belief exists everywhere, or that the principles I am suggesting are not already at least tacitly used. The existence of a hospice movement shows that there are other extant standards (even though hospice care is too infrequently available or used by the dying demented). I only want to note what appear to be the prevailing standards and why they need to be significantly modified in the case of those patients dying with dementia (though not uniquely with them).

There still remain some problems with the proposed criteria. The most obvious is in trying to determine when the time has come to invoke them: when is the deterioration sufficient to invoke the criteria? No precise moment can be specified; like much else in medicine it will be a matter of judgment. But some indicators can be suggested. One of them would be the emotional state of the patient. If there is evidence that the patient is suffering, whether evinced by the ordinary sounds of suffering (moaning, for instance) or by the body language of discomfort and agitated restlessness, then that apparent suffering should be taken seriously. If demented patients continue to have some kind of a self, they should be accorded all the usual deference given to someone who, apparently suffering, cannot verbally express himself. Thus evidence of suffering, verbal or nonverbal, should be a significant signal to terminate (or not to initiate) life-sustaining treatment.

Another indicator would be the degree of probability, based on clinical experience, that further treatment will enhance the likelihood of a poor death rather than an improved quality of life. Since this is a matter of probabilities, it will often not be easy to calculate. But, since the general course of dementia is downhill, there should be as much care to avoid increasing the odds of a poor death as care not to terminate treatment too quickly. Thus the standard for when the time has come to terminate treatment should not be set so high that the risk of a poor death is increased.[11]

## STIGMATIZATION AND ECONOMICS

I have sought here to find a middle way between the hazard of treating the demented too aggressively, as if their dementia counted for nothing in our judgment, and failing to give them sufficient treatment, on the grounds that their dementia removes them from the human community. The suggested standards for terminating treatment are meant to reassure those suffering from dementia in its early stages that we will not medically sustain their lives only to allow them a worse death; nor will we allow our horror of dementia to lead us to ignore or deny the self that may remain, even if damaged and all but hidden from our sight. I have looked for a stance that signals to demented patients and their families that we can and will terminate treatment if at all possible before total deterioration has taken place. But we will not do so in a way that suggests we have a special horror of the condition, creating criteria that allow us to stop treatment well before what would be acceptable with other patients. An approach of this kind could help to neutralize or at least reduce the hazard of stigmatization, which is likely to draw its force from a general dread of the disease exacerbated by policies suggesting the need to rush the demented out of their life and our midst. It may be hard to do much about the former, but we can at least ameliorate the potential hazards of the latter.

If for economic reasons it becomes necessary and desirable to give a low priority to the use of expensive life-extending technologies for late-stage terminal illness, including dementia, there is one place where a stronger stand should be taken. What does set dementia apart from other chronic and terminal illnesses is the impact upon families. Their lives can be crippled and harmed, even ruined, by the demands made upon them, at times cruel and inhuman. They need support of all kinds, economic and social and personal, and that costs money. If it is useless and wasteful and socially imprudent to extend marginally the life of the late-stage dementia patient, the same cannot be said of their families. Their lives will go on, and it is important that we help them to go on as well as possible.

## Acknowledgment

I want to thank The Greenwall Foundation for support of a project on Alzheimer disease at the Hastings Center.

## References

1. Ronald Dworkin, *Life's Dominion: An Argument About Abortion, Euthanasia, and Individual Freedom* (New York: Alfred A. Knopf, 1993), p. 195.
2. Sanford H. Radish, "Letting Patients Die: Legal and Moral Reflections," *California Law Review* 80 (1992): 857–888.
3. Joseph M. Foley, "The Experience of Being Demented," in *Dementia and Aging: Ethics, Values, and Policy Choices*, ed. Robert Binstock, Stephen Post, and Peter Whitehouse (Baltimore: The Johns Hopkins University Press, 1992), pp. 30–43.
4. Rebecca Dresser, "Missing Persons: Legal Perceptions of Incompetent Patients," *Rutgers Law Review* 46, no. 2 (1994): 690–719, at 690.
5. Tom Kitwood and Kathleen Bredin, "Toward a Theory of Dementia Care: Personhood and Weil-Being," *Ageing and Society* 12 (1992): 269–287.
6. Steven R. Sabat and Rom Harré, "The Construction and Deconstruction of Self in Alzheimer's Disease," *Ageing and Society* 12 (1992): 443–461.
7. Victoria Cotrell and Richard Schulz, "The Perspective of the Patient with Alzheimer's Disease: A Neglected Dimension of Dementia Research," *The Gerontologist* 33, no. 2 (1993): 206.
8. Richard C. Adelman, "The Alzheimerization of Aging," *The Gerontologist* 35, no. 4 (1995): 526–532.
9. Muriel R. Gillick, *Choosing Medical Care in Old Age: What Kind, How Much, Where to Stop* (Cambridge: Harvard University Press, 1994), p. 41.
10. Ladislav Volicer, Ann Collard, Ann Hurley, et al, "Impact of Special Care Unit for Patients with Advanced Alzheimer's Disease on Patients' Discomfort and Costs," *Journal of the American Geriatric Society* 42, no. 6 (1994): 597–603. See also Jill A. Rhymes and Laurence B. McCullough, "Nonaggressive Management of the Illnesses of Severely Demented Patients: An Ethical Justification," *Journal of the American Geriatrics Society* 42, no. 6 (1994): 686–687.
11. See Daniel Callahan, *The Troubled Dream of Life: In Search of a Peaceful Death* (New York: Simon & Schuster, 1993), pp. 187–219.

# 9

# KILLING AND ALLOWING TO DIE: WHY IT IS A MISTAKE TO DERIVE AN "IS" FROM AN "OUGHT"

Among most Anglo-American philosophers it has become settled dogma that there is no moral difference between killing a person directly (euthanasia) and terminating life-sustaining treatment (allowing to die)—and earlier called the difference between active and passive euthanasia. The philosopher James Rachels published an influential article in *The New England Journal of Medicine* in 1975, and it has been hard ever since to find any serious dissent, at least among philosophers (physicians seem to continue accepting the distinction).[1] The benefit of rejecting this distinction is that it more easily legitimates euthanasia. If it morally acceptable, for instance, to turn off the respirator of a dying patient—the claim goes—it should be no less acceptable to kill that patient directly (and perhaps more mercifully).

I can most easily present my argument against eliminating the distinction by offering an interpretation of three stages of life and death, both historically and in the life of a patient.

*Stage A: The healthy person and pre-modern medicine.* If there is no illness or disease, the human body functions well, requiring no medical support to remain alive. It is biologically self-sufficient. When that body became sick, however, pre-modern physicians could do no more than offer some diagnostic insight or advice on healthy living, unable to intervene effectively if illness struck. If the body was to heal, it had to heal itself. While there were rules against euthanasia and assisting a patient to commit suicide, there were no rules about the use of medicine to pre-serve life, which was beyond its power.

## Moral Rules Generated in Pre-Modern Medicine

—diagnosis when possible
—no euthanasia or physician-assisted suicide
—comfort to be given at all times

*Stage B: The onset of a lethal disease and the provision of life-extending treatment in modern medicine.* With the work of Francis Bacon and Rene Descartes in the 16th and 17th centuries, the idea of using scientific knowledge to cure illness and save life was introduced, even though it was then not actually possible to do so in a serious fashion. Medicine eventually moved on, making it possible by the mid-19th century to save and extend life, even if erratically. A new, second stage of care was introduced to the patient, accelerating by the end of that century and into the early 20th century. For the seriously ill patient hope became a realistic possibility. And when medicine historically reached that stage of its history, moral rules had to be constructed to deal with the new efficacy. I say "constructed" because neither medicine itself nor nature revealed any obvious guidance about what those rules should be. Rules were, however, devised over a period of time and are still in the process of construction as new technological possibilities and problems appear.

## Moral Rules Generated

—if life-extending treatments are available for otherwise lethal diseases, they should routinely be provided to patients if not unduly burdensome: doc-tors "ought" to provide life-extending treatment as a general rule.
—a doctor in such circumstances who does not provide treatment that could be efficacious, or who terminates treatment already begun in a similar cir-cumstance, is guilty of a serious moral wrong, the moral equivalent of directly killing the patient (and will be legally culpable for the omission). It was understood, however, that the patient died from the underlying ill-ness, not the cessation of treatment, whatever the physician's culpability.

*Stage C: When life-extending treatment proves futile, unduly burdensome, or is rejected by the patient.* This is the most recent historical stage where standard life-extending treatment, otherwise morally required, comes to appear questionable or wrong. Problems at this stage have become exacerbated because of the power of technology to extend failing life but often without providing more than marginal medical benefit, if any, and sometimes increasing the suffering of the patient. The ordinary treatment may seem futile in further arresting the lethal disease, physically or psychologically burdensome to the patient without corresponding benefit, or simply rejected by the (competent) patient.

## Moral Rules Generated

—it is morally wrong to deny a competent patient the right to refuse treatment, even if efficacious life-extending treatment

—it is morally acceptable for treatment to be terminated on an incompetent dying patient when the treatment is futile in arresting the course of the lethal disease, or when it is physically or psychologically an undue burden

—it is morally acceptable to use means of pain relief that run the *risk* of killing the patient, but not when they make certain the death of the patient (a form of euthanasia)

## THE ARTEFACTUAL FALLACY

I want now to explicate what I will call the "artefactual fallacy," by which I mean deriving an "is" from an "ought." A failure to take account of this fallacy, I believe, lies behind the judgment that there is no moral difference between killing and allowing to die. My contention is that, when treatment is stopped, the older view is correct: the patient is actually "killed" by the underlying lethal pathology, which has been temporarily arrested, not eliminated. The lethal disease, not the cessation of treatment, is the physical cause of death (as an autopsy would show). *It was only the construction of the moral rule positing an obligation to treat that allowed us to call a violation of that rule a culpable act and to treat it as if it was a form of direct killing and equivalent to the [physical] "cause" of death.* When that move is made, it then becomes easy to believe that there is no moral difference between killing and allowing to die—and no causal difference as well. The artefactual fallacy has been committed, usually unknowingly.

Let me provide a background defense of those assertions. The belief that it is not possible to derive an "ought" from an "is"—called the "naturalistic fallacy"— has been long accepted in moral philosophy (though dissenters can be found).

The way the world is does not tell us how we ought morally to respond to that world. Similarly, the fact that a person is biologically dying does not tell us how we ought to medically treat that patient—which is why moral rules had to be constructed when it became possible to provide life-extending treatment.

I want to define an "artefactual fallacy" as the opposite of the naturalistic fallacy: that of deriving an "is" from an "ought." The elimination of the distinction between killing and allowing to die commits this fallacy. It forgets that the rules concerning the cessation of treatment with dying patients are socially constructed rules, that is, moral artefacts that exist because humans invented, rather than discovered, them. When, therefore, it is argued that there is no difference between killing and allowing to die, a significant fact has been forgotten: that we have decided to act "as if" allowing a patient to die is a form of physical causation equivalent to directly killing a patient. But, biologically speaking, that is not true; it is only our constructed moral rule that makes it seem true. We have, that is, come to treat the "ought" as an "is," treating the moral rule as a biological fact in the world, not a moral construct.

What is a fact is that terminally ill patients whose lives have been medically extended live longer lives than those who have not had such treatment. They thus die at a later time than would otherwise be the case. If not killed directly, they will eventually die as a result of their (temporarily arrested) lethal disease either because treatment was stopped or because even the best available treatment no longer could stay the hand of death. If, during a blizzard, my driveway was filling with snow so rapidly that it was useless to continuing trying to shovel it, it would be a mistake to say that my failure to keep shoveling was the cause of the unstoppable snow filling the driveway and thus the equivalent of my shoveling snow into the driveway. Physicians who cannot stop death and cease treatment because of that cannot be said to be acting morally in the same way as a physician who directly kills a patient.

If my analysis is correct, then it also becomes wrong to claim that a physician who terminates treatment is, as a common phrase has it, "hastening" the death of the patient. A physician who has saved a patient from death at time "x," medically sustaining the life of the patient but unable to eliminate the underlying lethal pathology, cannot be accused of "hastening" death when, at a later elapsed time "y," he terminates life-extending treatment. The patient has already lived longer than if there had been no intervention in the first place. The overall course of dying has been slowed, and death cannot meaningfully said to be hastened if treatment is terminated after a significant period of time has passed between "x" and "y."

Here is an analogy. If, as a good swimmer, I see someone drowning, the moral rule in our society is that I ought to make every possible effort to save that person.

However, if I begin carrying that person into shore but eventually became unable to carry him any further, releasing him and thus allowing him to drown, I would not be accused of killing that person, even though it is the act of letting the person go that precipitates the final drowning. Nor would I be accused of "hastening" his death even if, had I tried, I might have carried him a few more meters. If, however, I deliberately let the drowning person go when I could easily have continued the rescue, then I would be held culpable for the act; and I could be treated "as if" I had killed that person. Either way, though, it is the water that biologically kills the drowning person, not my act of letting go.

Another example is relevant also. In his article James Rachels presents two cases, much cited thereafter, designed to show how the distinction between killing and allowing to die vanishes on closer examination:

"In the first [case], Smith stands to gain a large inheritance if anything should happen to his six-year-old cousin. One evening while the child is taking his bath, Smith sneaks into the bathroom and drowns the child, then arranges things so that it will look like an accident.

In the second [case], Jones also stands to gain if anything should happen to his six-year-old cousin. Like Smith, Jones sneaks in planning to drown the child in the bath. However, just as he enters the bathroom Jones sees the child slip and hit his head, and falls face down in the water. Jones is delighted; he stands by, ready to push the child's head back under if it is necessary, but it is not necessary. With only a little thrashing about, the child drowns all by himself, 'accidentally,' and Jones watches and does nothing."

In commenting on these two cases, Rachels says that "Now Smith killed the child, whereas Jones 'merely' let the child die. This is the only difference between them. Did either man behave better, from the moral point of view? If the difference between killing and letting die were in itself a morally important matter, one should say that Jones's behavior was less reprehensible than Smith's." Rachels denies, correctly, that Jones behaved less wrongly than Smith and contends, also correctly, that Jones could not get away with the defense that, concerning the child "'I didn't kill him; I only let him die.'"

There are two problems with this argument, one bearing on the meaning of the alleged moral equivalency of the two cases, the other bearing on the larger implications of Rachels's analysis for patient care and physician responsibility. On the first issue, the reason Rachels can contend that the moral blame is equal in both cases is that we have a social rule that, if one has a moral responsibility for the welfare of another, as an adult would for a six-year-old child, then a failure to save the life of such a child from drowning would make them culpable for a failure to do so. Smith would be morally culpable for killing the child, but Jones no less so for a failure to act when he should have. But there is a difference between killing and allowing to die in these cases. In the instance of Smith directly killing the child, the child dies because of the physical action of Smith; but for that action the child would still be alive. Jones, however, is not the physical cause of death, though because of our moral rules we hold him equally responsible for the death as if he had directly killed him.

Our moral rule in effect says that, in such situations, the actual physical cause of death is irrelevant; we have declared it so by virtue of our moral rule. But it is important to remember that the physical cause of death has not been abolished; it has been overlaid by a moral rule that declares it irrelevant. If, for instance, Jones had come upon a drowning insect in the bath tub and done nothing, we would have no hesitation in declaring the water as the cause of death and excused Jones of any responsibility. There is no rule of rescue with insects; we leave the insect's fate to nature.

The attribution of moral responsibility by means of a moral rule is, then, determinative of the moral significance of the actual physical cause of death. That conclusion becomes particularly important in the medical context. The Smith-Jones cases offer only a limited insight into medical decisions: we would have no trouble declaring immoral a doctor who turned off a respirator on a competent patient who wanted to be treated and one who, finding the respirator accidentally unplugged, decided not to plug it back in. That is hardly a common medical problem, at least as rare—and simple to solve morally—as the situation of Smith and Jones.

The full moral complexity for physicians arises when they have to decide whether the general moral rule to actively treat the critically ill and dying ought, because of the patient's medical status, to be set aside in favor of treatment termination and palliative care only. The current moral rule says that may be done if there is sufficient reason to do so. The question before us is whether, if a treatment termination is judged morally acceptable and the physician so acts, it can be said that the physician has acted no differently than if he had directly killed the patient by, say, an injection. My contention is that it is in most circumstances an entirely different act. It would only be similar if, for self-interested purposes, the physician terminated otherwise efficacious treatment in order to end the life of the patient—and even in that case it would be the underlying lethal disease that would be the necessary condition for such an action to kill the patient.

The truly pervasive problem for the physician has, at its core, a great puzzle and moral dilemma. On the one hand, nature has so ordered life biologically that, sooner or later, every patient will die. Unless we think that death is itself a biological accident, then one can add that not only *will* every patient eventually die, but every patient *must* die. At best the physician (or series of physicians, as the case may be) can only forestall death, not eliminate it. We will all die at some point but neither we nor our physicians know just when that will be.

On the other hand, the medical struggle consists of giving us as much time as possible, but only as long as that can be done without an undue burden of suffering. To properly treat the patient, then, the physician must be prepared to cease medically sustaining the patient when the treatment is no longer effective. If that is not done, the patient will eventually die anyway. But the patient, whose life has been artificially sustained, will die earlier than if that support had been continued. Yet the overriding reality is the inevitability of death. At stake is only its timing and circumstances, over which there can be some control. The moral debates have mainly turned on the issue of how much control under what circumstances to be determined by which persons.

One trend in recent decades has, seemingly, strengthened the contention that there is no moral difference between killing and allowing to die. It is that more and more lives, probably the majority, come to an end because of a decision to cease life-extending treatment. People do not, in other words, just die any more because of acts of nature but because of a decision to cease treating them, which will bring about death. It is human choice, not nature, which now ends most lives.

But that practice does not show that the killing-allowing to die distinction has been erased; the logical status of the distinction remains. But the practice might lead people to think, mistakenly, that nature no longer takes lives, only the actions of physicians. Except for the action of the physician in stopping treatment, the patient would have lived longer. Yet, in line with my earlier arguments, I would say that it is still the underlying disease that is the actual cause of death, not the physician's cessation of treatment. To change the timing, and only that, of an inevitable death from causes beyond the physician's control is not to kill the patient—even though it may appear that way to the outside observer. That observer has failed to note that we have come to think of treatment termination as the moral equivalent of killing, as if the physician was directly ending the patient's life. But it is only our socially constructed moral rule that treatment may, under certain circumstances, be terminated if various moral conditions have been met. The observer, in short, has committed the artefactual fallacy.

The artefactual fallacy then (a) treats our constructed moral rules as if they are biological facts, and (b) then equates them with direct killing, and (c) then holds that, morally speaking, there is no difference between killing and allowing to die. An "is" has thereby been derived from an "ought."

*Reference*

1. James Rachels, "Active and Passive Euthanasia," *The New England Journal of Medicine* 292:2 (January 9, 1975), pp. 78–80; for an interesting dissent (which seems to have made little difference with most philosophers), see Tom L. Beauchamp, "A Reply to Rachels on Active and Passive Euthanasia," in Tom L. Beauchamp and Seymour Perlin, eds., *Ethical Issues in Death and Dying* (Englewood Cliffs, N.J.: Prentice-Hall, 1978), pp. 246–258.

# 10

# RATIONING: THEORY, POLITICS, AND PASSIONS

A confession is in order. As did almost everyone else of a certain persuasion, I recoiled when Sarah Palin invoked the notion of a "death panel" to characterize reform efforts to improve end-of-life counseling. That was wrong and unfair. But I was left uneasy by her phrase. Had I not been one of a handful of bioethicists over the years who had pushed to bring the need for rationing of health care to public attention and proposed ways to carry it out? And was not a common thread running through the latter efforts the likely necessity of some kind of committee or other public mechanism to make the hard decisions? Were we not in other words talking about a "death panel," even if none of us has been so imprudent to use such a phrase? And did we not regularly bemoan the fact that politicians, left and right, would not go near the word "rationing"?

My answer to all those questions is yes, but with some important distinctions. One of them bears on the theoretical efforts to make a case for rationing and to propose means to carry it out. Another is the gap between that effort and the political realities of bringing rationing theory before the public eye. Still another is whether it is possible to envision an ethical theory that takes politics fully into account. But there is first a larger background story to be told about all that.

The larger story appropriately begins with the 1960 event that has often been thought of as the birth of bioethics. In that year, the University of Washington nephrologist Belding Scribner devised a shunt that would allow those suffering from kidney failure to be hooked up to a dialysis machine that could keep them alive for many years. But there were few of those machines and many more candidates for their use than could be accommodated. Rationing decisions of the most wrenching kind had to be made.[1]

The solution was a procedural one: the formation of two committees, one of them to determine the medical criteria for selecting candidates. The other was an Admissions and Policy Committee to choose, as the prominent journalist Shana Alexander wrote, "who shall live and who shall die." For four years that committee—whose membership was anonymous—made case-by-case decisions, and its general criterion was a troubling concept, that of the "social worth" of the patients. The committee had a dreadful time making such choices, and the very idea of such a committee was widely assaulted.

Dr. Scribner said later that "we had been naive" not to realize that what seemed to be the "reasonable and simple solution of…letting a committee of responsible members of the community choose patients" would evoke "a very serious storm of criticism."[2] Among those in ethics who entered the fray were James Childress and Paul Ramsey, who contended that a random lottery solution would be more fair, and the philosopher Nicholas Rescher, who favored a utilitarian solution that tacitly seemed to accept the "social worth" standard.

The dialysis controversy finally came to an end in 1972, when Congress passed a bill providing Medicare coverage for it. Money, in short, was the way out of the moral dilemmas of committee decisions. But why, many commentators asked, did Congress not do the same with lethal conditions such as cancer and heart disease? That question was answered with silence. Consistency is not one of the behavioral traits of Congress.

So far as I know, no similar effort to have committees make life and death decisions has ever been mounted in this country. Nonetheless, among those in bioethics who have written much on rationing over the years—Norman Daniels, Leonard Fleck, Paul Menzel, Alan Buchanan, Peter Ubel, and myself, for instance—there is a fair degree of consensus. I would sum it up as follows: if not at once, then sooner or later, rationing will be necessary (the steady rise of cost inflation will necessitate it); bedside rationing will not be acceptable (too open to bias and erratic criteria); rationing will have to be done at the policy level (mainly out of the hands of individual doctors and patients); and at that level there will have to be a decision-making procedure (most likely committees of some kind that will, with democratic deliberation, make transparent decisions with "accountability for reasonableness," to use Daniels's standard). The key point is that rationing decisions would be made at the policy level, not case by case.

I have left out most details with that list, as well as various disagreements among those who have written on rationing. Much of what we have written is theoretical in the sense that it has not been tested by much American experience—little save for Seattle is available—and makes ideal assumptions about ideal behavior in an ideally rational society.

But there is one European model that has been closely watched here, that of the United Kingdom's National Institute for Clinical Excellence (NICE). Technically, NICE was not established as a rationing agency—quality of care is its main emphasis—but it has the option of recommending to the British National Health Service that NHS not provide coverage for treatments thought to be of little medical value or judged to be too costly for their benefits. Most notable is its use of quality-adjusted life years (QALYs), an economics tool, to help it make decisions. The aim of that tool is to find a way around the subjectivity of decisions that will have to encompass individual quality-of-life judgments while at the same time not falling into the "social worth" swamp. The use of this tool is not meant to trump rational deliberation, but to supply it with an economic criterion, recognizing that it would inevitably have some value considerations. It was, not surprisingly, singled out for particular condemnation by opponents of the reform legislation, a this-could-happen-to-us menace if we are not vigilant.

The recent and no doubt endless health care reform debate in the United States was a shock to many of us who have toiled in the neatly tilled vineyard of rationing theory. At first all looked well. Fully recognized was the reality of unsustainable cost escalation with its fallout of a growing number of uninsured, excessive out-of-pocket expenses, Medicaid crises in most states, and a projected insolvency of Medicare in seven to eight years. The Democratic leadership, with at least initial Republican support, made perfectly clear that strong steps to control costs would be necessary.

But as time went on, the expected fast-track drive to manage costs became more a soft, slow, decade-long shuffle. Nervousness about the subject of costs was perfectly exemplified in President Obama's assurance that there would be no reduction of Medicare benefits for seniors. I have seen no serious analysis of Medicare's future that does not include just such a reduction to remain sustainable. "Bending the curve" became the anodyne term of choice in light of the political reality that rapid, fast options would not make it.

Perhaps the reform legislation will make a long-term difference, but even if it does, there is some consensus that it will not do what is necessary: bringing annual cost escalation in line with the annual rise of the gross domestic product, from the present 6% to 3%. The costs of care for the baby boomers about to enter the Medicare program by the millions will be staggering. Many astute policy analysts have long noted that, for Medicare to survive, either a doubling of the tax rate or a 50% cut in benefits will be necessary. No one talks that way in Congress.

Nor does the reform legislation do much to stem the steady stream of expensive biologic drugs for cancer care and costly medical devices for heart disease, many of which cry out for some rationing. How many new cancer drugs costing between fifty and one hundred thousand dollars for just a few extra months of life can be afforded? The stipulation in the reform legislation that comparative effectiveness research could be used neither to fashion practice guidelines nor even to make recommendations for the use of its findings was as good a sign as any that cost control would not encompass directly saying no to patients, doctors, or industry. Pressures from the drug and device industries and some physician groups were responsible for that crippling provision.

If end-of-life care as legislatively envisioned was the wrong place to affix the label of "death panels," Sarah Palin surely had a good nose for the political unacceptability of any rationing talk. Republicans fastened unrelentingly on any whiff of it (particularly exploiting slippery slope arguments), and Democrats shied away from it no less persistently. What candidate for reelection will go home admitting to his elderly constituents that he favors a cut in their benefits? Far from opening the door for some serious discussion of rationing, it was slammed shut in the reform run-up.

Most of the assumptions about the value and plausibility of deliberative democracy (bringing the public into direct engagement) that have been a key part of the theoretical rationing ensemble have been rendered inoperable. Too many people seem to want no deliberation of any kind. How can we have a sensible public discussion of panels making use of "accountability for reasonableness" if perhaps half of our fellow citizens consider it immoral even to talk about it? Putting aside the often hostile hysteria that marked any efforts to even raise the topic, it is not hard to discern the roots of the opposition. There is the deeply embedded hostility to government interference in the doctor-patient relationship—assumed to be a bulwark against rationing—financially well supported by many medical groups and the drug and device industry. Then there is the popular expectation that in principle the benefits of medical progress and health care should be available to everyone regardless of costs. That view is held by many physicians and encouraged by a research enterprise ever ready to trumpet its benefits, that of the decisive nostrums and cures just over the next hill. That public expectation is not matched by a willingness to pay for the promised benefits, but it is strong enough to stifle any talk of limits to care.

Most important, perhaps, is the belief that, in a rich country like ours, the money is really out there to pay for all we want or need. Liberals can point to the billions spent on unnecessary wars or agricultural subsidies. Conservatives claim that the problem is a failure to let the market, with its potentially rich mix of private choice and insurer competition, be given its unregulated head. Again and again, moreover, I have found it possible with some patience to persuade all but the fanatical in some general fashion that some rationing, in some way, at some time or other, will be necessary, only to be told, "Yes, you're right, but not if it is my spouse, child, or grandparent." For them, the moral bottom line is that rationing life and death is intrinsically wrong, and the test case is someone they cherish.

Nor is that just an American problem. In sketching the earlier cited consensus among the bioethicists who have worked on rationing, I left out the agreement that fair rationing could take place only in a universal health care system, one with equal access to care and (I would add) a fixed annual budget. That would force tradeoffs in the face of scarcity and allow consideration of the opportunity costs of different rationing possibilities.

The United Kingdom has such a health care system, and in NICE it has a way of doing some rationing. But does that combination save it from the kind of politics that stifle debate here? Possibly a little, but not entirely by any means. While there have been critics of NICE's methodology, including its use of QALYs, they have been matched by complaints that its deliberations are not sufficiently transparent, particularly among the subcommittees that carry out most of them. That may well be true about the process, but the recommendations, and the NHS role in responding to them, make their way to the public by means of an ever-alert, aggressive media. The NHS is obliged to cover those treatments and technologies that meet the NICE standards (one reason why these treatments often raise costs), but its conclusions about covering treatments that fall short of the standards can be made only as recommendations.

Recommendations against coverage (or to limit coverage) of some expensive drugs for cancer and dementia on grounds of their high cost per QALY have caught the eye of the media—and the British media is far more unbuttoned than its American counterpart. Its reporters typically fan out to interview those who will be denied a drug. For cancer patients, that drug will often extend their lives, even if not for long. No less typically, those denied the drug or their families believe the drug has desirable benefits (never mind what unseen experts say) and that it would be inhumane to put a price tag on their lives. Why inflict that nastiness on them? This equals a perfect tabloid story. As Robert Steinbrook noted in a paper on NICE, "After all, saying no takes courage—and inevitably provokes outrage."[3]

Ironically, then, transparency can turn out to make rationing decisions all the more difficult to implement. As a result of public outcries, a number of NICE recommendations against coverage have been taken to court, and the NHS has had to back down on some that it initially accepted. Efforts to include more patients in NICE's rationing deliberations may well exacerbate that result. As two advocates for that shift put it, the economic techniques used by NICE "do not measure the quality of someone's life in a way that is sensitive to a variety of conditions or that allows individuals to indicate what is important to them personally and how their illness affects that. …Although the direct costs of some treatments may place a huge burden on society, rationing such treatments places even greater (indirect) costs on individuals, their careers, and the wider population."[4]

The logic of that kind of individual patient variation argument is but a short step to a Seattle-type committee, with case-by-case decisions. It also has a more recent familiar ring: U.S. opponents of evidence-based guidelines based on population statistics have said much the same thing. They conclude that it would be better to leave all final decisions in the hands of doctors and their patients, not government panels peopled by faceless bureaucrats. A sick person's notion of "accountability for reasonableness," much less the results of even full democratic deliberation, may offer little solace to someone deprived of a longer (even if not much longer) or in their eyes better life, however awful it might seem in ours.

Yet however much individual patients may be hurt or aggrieved by rationing decisions, they will have to be made eventually. They will have to be a main, if hardly the only, ingredient in any long-term solution to the cost escalation problem—a problem that has the potential to wreak economic and medical havoc if not taken more seriously. It is the classic and always difficult dilemma of individual versus common good. To make matters worse, we do not ordinarily attribute a desire to live rather than die, or to feel less pain rather than more, to gross selfishness. In the case of just wars, we are prepared to sacrifice our children to defend us from societal ruin—but only when there is no other choice. But in the case of health care rationing, it has proved nearly impossible to have a serious debate about something many consider a prima facie evil. As in the United Kingdom, the American media would instantly seize upon the predictable moral outrage.

It is harder still to cut through the plethora of upbeat ideas to avoid rationing, starting with those old nostrums: first, the assertion that we need no rationing until we have eliminated all waste and inefficiency in our health care system or carried out more and better research to rid us of all those expensive diseases; or second—all other ideas failing—the assertion that it does not matter what we spend on health care, held by some economists to be the best possible way to spend money (even in a severe recession, health care remains one of the few economic domains that regularly adds jobs).

Is there some way to develop a theory of rationing that takes full account of the political turbulence of heath care reform and the deep repugnance felt by many, maybe even most, at the possibility of rationing? None that I have heard of. If politics has made it hard to manage in the United Kingdom, with its tradition of more readily accepting health care limits than the United States has, it seems almost insurmountable in our hyperindividualistic culture, suffused with skepticism about, or outright hostility to, a strong role for government and an excessively great love of new, always better, technologies.

I find it plausible to think of rationing in three categories. One of them I call "direct and naked": an unveiled denial of some important health benefit, including life-extending treatment, by either a private or public institution that has the power to do so. To be sure, there is a great difference between rationing in the context of absolute shortages, as with the early dialysis machines, and denying the sick an insurance or Medicare benefit, but leaving them free to buy it for themselves. The latter will be small comfort for anyone other than the very affluent; many families bankrupt themselves these days to cover treatments they cannot otherwise afford.

By "indirect and veiled" rationing, I have in mind the use of copayments and deductibles, particularly when they are set high enough to discourage but not to openly stop people from using expensive services. By "covert" rationing, I mean the kind that existed in the United Kingdom from the 1950s through at least the early 1980s. Restrained by tight budgets, it came to be understood as an unwritten rule that patients over the age of fifty-five would be denied dialysis and some forms of heart surgery. They were to be told by their physicians that nothing could be done for them. That was a flat lie, but it offered cover to physicians who knew their limited budgets could not stand it.

The eminent British policy analyst Rudolf Klein has suggested that a less visible form of that earlier practice still exists in the United Kingdom: "the most pervasive form of rationing is the least explicit and least visible: rationing by dilution...not to order an expensive diagnostic test, or to reduce ward staffing levels in order to balance the budget normally attract little attention unless they explode in a scandal...such decisions are as much a form of rationing as the refusal to prescribe a drug...however, in the times ahead no generally accepted decision-making model is likely to emerge." "The best that ministers can hope for," Klein concludes, "is that most rationing will continue to take the form of dilution rather than excision and that decisions can be taken in the name of clinical discretion and thus be politically invisible."[5]

If present ethical theories—not designed for nasty fights—will not help or be much listened to, just what might otherwise happen? I would bet on a combination of gradually increased taxes, an expanded government role despite conservative hostility, and a steady, even accelerating, rise of co-payments, deductibles, and coinsurance—already a pervasive practice. Will there be complaints? Of course. But a long-losing Yale football coach once said that the trick with the alumni was to "keep them sullen, but not mutinous." Copayments and deductibles have managed to walk that fine line. They will surely continue to rise and are steadily doing so across Medicare, Medicaid, and private insurance.

While covert rationing will undoubtedly be condemned, I would not be surprised if it starts happening. For at least some physicians, it will be an enticing way of dealing with cost pressures, a kind of well-meant falsehood to avoid the pain of brutal candor. Available information in the media and on the Internet will make it much harder now to get away with that tactic, but since patients tend to trust their doctors, some doctors may succeed. Rudolf Klein's dour but sober judgment of rationing in the United Kingdom may, and probably will, be applicable here as well.

The rationing problem in the end is that we have a culture and politics that invite evasion of hard ethical dilemmas, outrage and shouting instead of deliberative democracy, and a bad case of what has been called "the California disease"—a limit on taxation combined simultaneously with unlimited demands for ever-more benefits. We want unbounded medical progress, an all-out war on death, lower taxes, and no medical rationing. It is a mix that cannot long be sustained but, like a drug-resistant virus, it continues mutating to keep us sick. It is a chronic economic disease as tenacious as the medical ones. No less pathological is an unwillingness on the part of politicians to talk openly about the need for rationing, not just what's wrong with it. Euphemisms, evasions, and rosy scenarios of bending the curve, or of simultaneously improving quality while lowering costs, make up the rhetoric of choice.

The culture of evasion directly clashes with the necessity of cost control. The same political forces clamoring for deficit reduction are those that have most vehemently condemned any talk of rationing. They cannot have it both ways. Something has to give. But there is little reason to think that what gives will be evasion. I find it hard to imagine that open rationing will be possible other than with the low-hanging fruit—whatever is the least threatening and economically marginal. The really hard choices will be pushed into the territory of indirect and covert rationing. The reigning ethical theory on rationing has it right: only committee decisions with considerable public input ought to be acceptable. But that model has not yet been taken seriously in the world of politics—a failure that simply increases the likelihood that ethically flawed strategies will be embraced. That will be a shame.

*References*

1. A.R. Jonsen, *The Birth of Bioethics* (New York: Oxford University Press, 1998), 211 ff; R.C. Fox and J.P. Swazey, *Courage to Fail: A Social View of Organ Transplants and Dialysis* (Chicago, Ill.: University of Chicago Press, 1974).

2. Quoted in Fox and Swazey, *Courage to Fail*, 76.

3. R. Steinbrook, "Saying No Isn't NICE—The Travails of Britain's Institute for Health and Clinical Excellence," *New England Journal of Medicine* 359 (2008): 1981.

4. J. Speight and M. Reaney, "Wouldn't It Be NICE to Consider Patient's Views When Rationing Health Care," *British Medical Journal* 338 (2009): b85.

5. R. Klein, "Rationing in the Fiscal Ice Age," *Health Economics, Policy and Law* 5, no. 4 (2010): 389–396, at 389–390 and 394.

# 11

# CONSUMER-DIRECTED HEALTH CARE: PROMISE OR PUFFERY?

It is probably no accident that one of the leading American enthusiasts for consumer-directed health care (CDHC), Regina Herzlinger, is a faculty member at the Harvard Business School. Not only does she draw her model of health care directly from the business community, she also touts it with all the verve of a campaign worked up by the school's marketing department: "The US health care system is in the midst of a ferocious war...a system controlled by the insurance companies or hospitals or government will kill us financially and medically...there is only one group that can prevent this damage: consumers—you and me—working together with our doctors" (Herzlinger, 2007: 1). It is probably no accident either that consumer-directed health care seems to be an excessively American idea, a combination of our distrust of government, our hyper-individualism, and our love of the market. Nonetheless, other countries I gather are flirting with the idea in one form or another.

I cite Herzlinger because she is one of CDHC's more colorful and prominent proponents, particularly in the pages of influential newspapers such as *The Wall Street Journal*. That paper is one of the strongest supporters of George W. Bush's campaign to privatize as much of America's health care as possible, and consumer-directed health care is one of the leading means of doing so. While it is possible to separate the politics of consumer-directed health care from its economic substance, as I will shortly try to do, that combination has given it more public clout than economics alone.

If the economic aim of CDHC is to empower patients to be thoughtful consumers, its political aim is to move American health care away from a fee-for-service model. That model encourages patients to be ignorant of and indifferent to costs. CDHC will force them to make sensible choices based on value for money—their money, and not that of government or insurers. CDHC rests on the premise that health care can successfully be treated the same as other commodities, that patients should be free to choose their own form of health care, and that they should be able to select from among robustly competitive private-sector insurers.

If those goals can be accomplished, the argument goes, the result will be a high-quality, economically efficient system. That promissory note is for many most appealing, particularly at a time when almost all observers, not to mention the general public, believe the American health care system is in deep trouble, beset by some 47 million uninsured and by a 7% annual cost inflation rate, projected to double in a decade or so. I will focus on the American scene, not only because I know it better but also because, though relatively new, it has been studied and analyzed. I will not take up another form of medical care, also called consumer-directed, which has been embraced to improve long-term care for the elderly and younger people with disabilities. Its aim is better self-care and integration of care services and it does not focus on cost control or overall health care reform as the mainline CDHC does. It is sometimes known as the "independent living model," and has been taken up in Austria, Germany, and The Netherlands (Kodner, 2003). The premise CDHC embraces is a direct rejection of the much-cited argument advanced by the Nobel laureate Kenneth Arrow in his 1963 article "Uncertainty and the Welfare Economics of Health Care" (Arrow, 1963). Health care, he contended, is different from other areas of economic activity, presenting many features that make a good medical market hard to achieve. The nature of demand for health care is "irregular and unpredictable"; the patient is forced to trust his physician, lacking the latter's knowledge and experience; the customer "cannot test the product before using it"; "recovery from disease is as unpredictable as its incidence"; and entry into the field of health care is limited by professional and licensing restrictions.

For many years there was little opposition within health care economics to Arrow's thesis. Long afterwards, however, in a special issue of the *Journal of Health Care, Policy and Politics* devoted to Arrow's work, James C. Robinson sharply broke ranks by writing that "the most pernicious doctrine in health services research, the greatest obstacle to clear and successful action, is that health care is *different...* To some within the health care community, the uniqueness doctrine is self-evident and needs no justification" (Robinson, 2001: 1045). To judge health care "different" is to block many management techniques that could be effectively used in health care organization.

Supporters of CDHC agree with Robinson's judgment but came to it on their own, stimulated by the success of the market-oriented business community. That community has thrived on consumer choice and commercial competition, and it has improved quality and lowered costs for its products, stimulated innovation and raised everyone's standard of living. What better model for emulation could there possibly be? Translated into the lay vernacular, "consumer-directed health care supposes a new formulation—one driven by consumers with cash-in-hand, demanding to know for themselves who is the best urologist in town, what are my treatment alternatives, why is this hospital billing so much for a Tylenol, why can't I read this prescription, where is the nurse when I need one, how do I get the most value for the money I'm spending?" (Scandlen, 2004: 1117). As that quotation suggests, it will be perfectly appropriate for those consumers (once known as patients) to be demanding, insistent, impatient, carping, and Scrooge-like when double-checking their hospital bill for Tylenol charges.

I will turn to a more formal examination of CDHC, without the vivid color and heated enthusiasm, often evangelical in flavor, which many of its proponents display. A good place to start is with a more technical definition of what CDHC is, and this one is useful: "Many would agree that the term generally refers to a health benefit design where consumers have a high deductible insurance plan, a personal account funded in various ways to pay for care, a gap between the annual amount put into the account, and an internet-based decision support system" (Clancy and Gauthier, 2004: 1049). By a "high deductible" is typically meant $1,000 or more. There are two forms of such plans, a health savings account (HSA) and a health reimbursement arrangement (HRA). The former allows employees to put money, tax free, into a savings account, and to take money out. Also required, however, is a parallel insurance policy to cover catastrophic costs, which is where the high deductible comes into play. An HRA by contrast is an employer-funded savings account to achieve the same end, but will not necessarily require a parallel catastrophic insurance policy.

Now assuming that a British or European reader can make sense of all this— which so far as I know has no parallel in their health care systems (and which is relatively new for Americans as well)—the story is actually a bit more complicated than I have so far implied. Regina Herzlinger, for instance, celebrates the great possibilities of consumer choice and savvy, of a kind they display when buying automobiles and cell phones. Once free from the grip of academic elites, government, insurance companies, hospitals, and sometimes even doctors, they will make good choices and, along the way, force providers to do a better job. But a Harvard Business School colleague, Michael E. Porter, is co-author of a book that is skeptical of overly strong claims about consumer sovereignty: a patient's relationship with his doctor is not the same as with an auto salesman (Porter and

Teisberg, 2006). Their contention is that the key to a more robust system is com-petition for value; that is, the quality of health outcomes. They support CDHC, but say that it cannot achieve its potential in the face of dysfunctional competi-tion, by which he means competition to shift costs, to increase bargaining power, to capture patients and restrict choice, and to reduce costs by reducing services. They call those tactics "zero-sum" competition (Porter and Teisberg, 2006: 35).

An interesting exchange in *Health Affairs* in 2006 brought out some variants on the nature and aims of CDHC. The lead article, focused primarily on costs and quality, presented a consumer-oriented emphasis "to provide consumers with incentives to use care wisely and shop for high-value services" (Buntin *et al.*, 2006: w516). But each of the three respondents to the article had a different inter-pretation of its aims and significance. One of them argued that the emphasis on consumers was too narrow. The broader problem is the need for "quality-based benefit design," and said that to shift costs to consumers is a "threat to access and evidence-based medicine." Moreover, there is now an expectation that all health plans provide good patient information and support.

Another respondent, Tony Miller, a cofounder of Definity Health, one of the earliest consumer-directed health plans, rejects the view that CDHC is just a way of shifting costs to consumers and helping them to make "rational economic deci-sions" (Miller, 2006: w549). It is instead "about a change in the way we are going to finance our consumption of health care services so that users of those serv-ices have more control over how the dollars are spent." The third respondent, John Goodman, contends that CDHC is essentially a rationing device to stem an unsustainable rise in health care costs, a disastrous trajectory. In the end, it will be patients themselves who must make the hard choices "between health care and other uses of money...[and] it is appropriate and desirable for people to make these decisions themselves—and to reap the full benefits and bear the full costs of their decisions" (Goodman, 2006: w540–w541). Goodman well articulates—but favorably so—just that view which those suspicious of the motives behind the rise of CDHC hold: that HSAs are a "small but important step in the direction of a health care system in which individuals ration their own health care, instead of having those decisions made by impersonal bureaucracies or doctors who answer to those bureaucracies."

Those variant interpretations of the meaning and direction of CDHC force a consideration of the role that politics and ideology play in its promotion. From President Bush down through conservative and Republican ranks, the specter of "socialized medicine" is the political goad to keep the US from moving in the direction of a government-run or regulated universal health care system, about which enough bad things cannot be said. While proponents of CDHC surely share that bias, most agree that there must be a government role to care for the poor and the elderly; but, beyond that safety net, the less government the better. Patient choice and provider competition for everyone else is made to order from that perspective, and the much celebrated private sector—held up as a model of efficiency, quality and cost control—provides a template to make it all work.

That much said, the language of politics and ideology is more observable in the public media and in conservative blogs than it is among health care economists and professional health policy analysts. The latter have brought to bear their technical skills to examine the CDHC phenomenon, both favorably and unfavorably. Almost all of them make a point of noting that it is a movement and set of ideas that have not been around long enough for any definitive judgment; the "jury is still out" is a common phrase. And as might be expected there is a range of tentative judgments, primarily bearing on the control of costs, quality, patient, and employer satisfaction, and the likely future of CDHC.

The focus of analysis has primarily been on four issues: the extent of growth and popularity of CDHC, its impact on costs and quality, its potential for inequity, and the possibility of meaningful patient choice. Almost everything we know comes out of CDHC's early days, and a new round of studies of more recent developments have yet to appear.


## EXTENT OF GROWTH AND POPULARITY OF CDHC

Despite earlier expectations that CDHC plans would grow rapidly, that has not happened. As of 2006, only about 4% of eligible employees were enrolled in such plans, about the same as the previous year. Employers from large businesses were more likely to offer such plans, but they do not have much hope that such plans will reduce costs. While there has been a fair degree of patient satisfaction with the CDHC, the reports on the availability of the information they need to make good choices has sometimes been difficult to find (Christianson *et al.*, 2004; Fowles *et al.*, 2004).


## IMPACT ON COST AND QUALITY

Despite employer skepticism about cost reductions from CDHC programs, at least two studies found there were some (Gabel *et al.*, 2004). One of them was particularly optimistic, finding that costs in their study were lower and achieved without a negative impact on health (Bertko, 2004). Another found that, while costs were lower, participants had a higher rate of resource intensive hospital care (for reasons that were unclear) (Parente, 2004). Still another study concluded that lower costs and lower cost increases were achieved, though the specific magnitude was not specified. But the evidence on improvement of quality was mixed (Buntin *et al.*, 2006). One commentator noted that various studies ranged from the somewhat unfavorable to the highly favorable, indicating that context, location, and different plan designs led to different responses. But for him that poses no problem: market plans (unlike those set by government) are open to change and correction (Scandlen, 2004). Everything can be altered and improved in the market; like the famous river of the ancient philosopher Heraclitus, one never steps twice in the ever-changing market.

George C. Halvorson, however, is exceedingly skeptical that CDHR can achieve any significant cost savings: CDHC plans allow their participants to use the money available to them from their medical savings account to pay those costs they choose to pay by deciding to obtain or not obtain possible health care. But this will only make sense with low-cost treatments, and those are not the important costs. It was known long ago that co-payments and deductibles will lower health care utilization, but, for the most critical illnesses, they make no difference. As Halvorson reminds us (of something known, but usually ignored), "The vast majority of people use almost no care. Seventy percent of the population, in fact, use less than 10% of all care dollars, and 5% use an absolute majority of all money spent on care" (Halvorson, 2004: 1119).

## POTENTIAL FOR INEQUITY

A persistent worry from the outset of CDHC has been its potential for inequity (Bloche, 2006). Would it attract only the well and the affluent, not the sick and the poor, and craftily shift costs from employers to employees? It is hard to imagine a more harsh evaluation of the meaning of CDHC than the following: "Driven by a philosophy that favors unbridled faith in the free marketplace, the year 2003 may well go down in health care history as the year that the health care system officially abandoned the premise that a community has a responsibility to care for each member, replacing it with the philosophy that individuals should each look after themselves" (Shearer, 2004: 1159).

The reference is to the passage by Congress of the Medicare Prescription Drug Improvement and Modernization Act of 2003, an Act that was President Bush's most important effort to privatize more of American health care. In addition to providing prescription drug coverage for the elderly for the first time (much to the irritation of some even more zealous market proponents), it also set in place HSAs, an important stimulant for CDHC. For supporters of universal health care, that was an important setback and obviously, for Shearer, a symbol of a disastrous downward slide. And we might recall that Dr John Goodman, cited above, thinks that is just fine.

The reality so far seems far less disastrous than Shearer imagined. The slowness with which CDHC is being taken up, the mixed reports on whether it attracts only the affluent and the healthy (though the general trend has been that it disproportionately attracts high-income and high-status employees), suggests it is neither going to be as bad as some think nor as much of a help to American health care as its supporters hope. Karen Davis, President of the Commonwealth Fund, concluded that the HSR study I have frequently cited, suggested that CDHC did not show great promise for major health reform: "Consumer-directed health care—if it is primarily a tool for shifting costs from employers to employees—will quickly be discredited. A strategy aimed primarily at providers to identify, demand, and reward high performance, with positive incentives for consumers in a complementary role, is likely to have greater long-term success and adaptability" (Davis, 2004: 1230).

## THE PROBABILITY OF INFORMED PATIENT CHOICES

Two notes that rarely get struck in the debate on CDHC are those of medical uncertainty and medical probabilities. They are central realities in clinical medicine. In a large number of cases, the proper treatment of patients is uncertain and the outcome of those treatments is no less uncertain. In equally large numbers, almost everything in diagnosis and just about everything in treatment outcomes is a matter of probabilities as well. Doctors are often uncertain because a knowledge of the general probabilities of a particular course of treatment is not a certain predictor of what will work with individual patients. The uncertainties and probabilities become all the more common, and perplexing, with critically ill patients suffering from multi-organ failure, often the most expensive patients and prime consumers of ICU beds and intensive treatment time. CDHC supporters pass too easily over these everyday complexities.

If doctors have trouble diagnosing and treating patients, a much-cited study of cost-sharing by patients carried out by the Rand Corporation and directed by Joseph Newhouse in the early 1970s (well before the CDHC era) showed that, in making cost-sharing decisions, patients can make wrong as well as right choices (Newhouse, 1993). An important aim of the study, conducted as an experiment, was to test the economic theory that patient cost sharing reduced health care services; and that turned out to be true. But if in general there were no significant harms from using fewer services, patients also had no good way of distinguishing between care that was needed and care that was not needed. Moreover, the poor were more likely to delay getting treatment than the better off, incurring later harm. Many contemporary proponents of CDHC would respond that greater transparency, more information, and patient education can reduce that hazard, but that remains to be seen.

A more fundamental problem is the assumption that, properly equipped with savvy and information, patients can make their way through the health care system. But it is striking that the complexity of many medical decisions is scanted in the CDHC literature. The working premise seems to be that new and modernized patients will be of full mental capacity, rational in all things, saturated with the latest and best information culled from the best internet guides, and tough enough to fight their way past paternalistic doctors and slow-moving nurses to get their own way.

Consider a real life person: me. Trained as a philosopher I am a professionally certified rationalist. And as someone who spends his time in medical circles, I think I am reasonably well-situated and sophisticated enough to be an ideal consumer. Recently, I was put to a test, one that my older male readers will recognize. My physician discovered an elevated prostate-specific antigen (PSA) score (a possible symptom of prostate cancer), and one that was rapidly rising over a short time. He quickly and repeatedly insisted that I was free to make my own choice about further treatment. He recommended a biopsy, but along the way I had discovered that some urologists think PSA tests are so unreliable they personally refuse to take them. Others believe that, as someone past 75, there is not much point in taking one anyway, and even less point in having a follow-up biopsy. Since I am 77, I felt that for once old age was a blessing, sparing me the need for a biopsy. But I also discovered that by no means do all physicians accept that limit.

The more I read the more uncertain I became about what to do, and the more I pressed my physician and other medical colleagues the more it all came down to probabilities, and different clinicians often attach different meanings to the same probabilities. You are not necessarily going to die, I was reassured to hear, but "you are at increased risk," a phrase I could get no doctor to attach a number to. But in the end, I did what many others do in a similar situation: I did what my physician recommended and had the biopsy. He had, after all, treated many patients with potential or actual prostate cancer. He had experience and I did not, and I was in no position to judge among the warring factions on the treatment of that disease. The biopsy was negative, which was a good thing. The medical disputes about how best to treat prostate cancer are even more controversial than whether to get screened for it in the first place. The urologist who performed the biopsy asked me to come back for another blood test in six months. A year has passed, and I have not done so, nor do I intend to do so. I started out as a self-directed consumer and ended as a defeated consumer.

I am certain most readers of this paper, either through personal experience or that of family or friends, can tell a story of medical uncertainties in treating serious conditions. As my wife, suffering once from some obscure long condition, observed "modern medicine is just wonderful but less good with whatever your personal illness happens to be." An exaggeration perhaps, but not by much. Paul Ginsburg, an economist and President of the Center for Studying Health System change, has written "to pretend that consumers alone can transform our complex, fragmented system is naive at best and disingenuous at worst. Current efforts to increase price transparency often downplay the difficulty of medical decisions, patient's dependence on physicians for treatment guidance, and the need for meaningful information on quality" (Ginsburg, 2007).

Ginsburg does not deny the benefit of choosing providers that offer better values and agrees that some market pressures will lead providers to improve their performance on both cost and quality. But, unlike much writing on CDHC, there is some important clinical realism that he reminds us makes the purchase of health care far more complicated than buying a car or refrigerator. I might observe as well that, if there came to be many consumers of the obnoxious kind described above by Scandlen (2004), physicians and nurses would be sorely tempted to prematurely pull out a few tubes and turn off some respirators to shut them up. Fortunately, I would surmise that patients with any common sense would determine that getting one's doctors and nurses angry is not a good idea. Our car dealer has no power over us, but however sophisticated we may be about the kind of care we want, we cannot get rid of the fact that doctors and nurses have more power over us than we do over them.


## CONSUMER-DIRECTED HEALTH CARE: PROMISE OR PUFFERY?

I believe a distinction can be made between patients who inform themselves about the best available physicians, hospitals, and clinics, who try to educate themselves about the choices they will have to make, economic and medical, and who expect their reasonable wishes to be honored—and those who embrace CDHC in its most ambitious reform models. The former should also be wise enough to know that medical care is filled with uncertainties, that they will have to trust their physicians, and that things can turn out poorly, and go from bad to worse. The commercial model of health care, extrapolated from the commercial sector has some severe limits. A new model is undoubtedly coming into being, still in the making, the result of better-educated patients, a gradual change in the once wholly paternalistic doctor–patient relationship, and in the information available to patients.

But there remains an irreducible and eventually inevitable part of the medical experience. We will at some point, and perhaps often, be weak and uncertain, not at our rational best, not knowing what to make of the information we receive (almost guaranteed with any serious illness to be conflicting, one group of experts rejecting another, leaving us at sea). As we get older, and more of our organs start falling apart, our brains if not demented just a bit fuzzier, our vulnerability, our human finitude will increasingly assert itself. The smart consumer, the good shopper, the self-confident directed autonomous self will fade away, nostalgically longed for but no longer present. Consumer-directed health care appears to be a good fair-weather friend, up to dealing with a small squall, but not really bad weather.

I have said little about health care competition other than to cite the work of Porter and Teisberg (2006). Consumer-directed health care, to be successful in controlling costs, must give patients a competitive range of choice on the price of care, where they receive it, their physicians, and its quality. Otherwise, choice becomes meaningless. At least in the United States competition in the private sector has not been able to control costs (now increasing at a rate of 7% a year) and, given the likelihood that if CDHC does have some success in controlling costs, it will be at the margins, not in critical care medicine where the heaviest costs appear.

Nor can one ignore an international phenomenon: health care and competition are always likely to be more robust in densely crowded urban areas than in distant suburbs or rural settings. In the latter areas, there will be fewer doctors to choose among, and fewer hospitals and clinics available. There is no obvious way to overcome disparities of this kind, at least none in any country I have heard of (ask the Canadians, Alaskans, and Swedes about achieving equitable care near the Arctic Circle). Small, scattered communities are not places rich in doctors to choose among or in hospitals to provide care. As Henry Ford once remarked of his model T: "You can have any color you like as long as it is black." That's as close as many people will get to meaningful choice and competition in health care.

Consumer-directed health care: promise or puffery? A little of both but more puffery than promise.

*References*

Arrow, K. (1963), "Uncertainty and the welfare economics of health care," *American Economic Review*, 53: 941–973.

Bertko, J. (2004), "Commentary-looking at the effects of consumer-centric health plans on expenditures and utilization," in Clancy and Gauthier (eds), *Health Services Research (HSR)*, 39(4): 1211–1218.

Bloche, M. (2006), "Consumer-directed health care," *The New England Journal of Medicine,* 357(17): 1756–1759.

Buntin, M.B., C. Damberg, A. Haviland, K. Kapur, N. Lurie, R. McDevitt, and M.S. Marquis (2006), "Consumer-directed health care: early evidence about effects on cost and quality," *Health Affairs*—Web exclusive, Special Supplement, Part II, 25(6): W516-W530.

Christianson, J., S. Parente, and R. Feldman (2004) "Consumer experiences in a consumer-driven health plan," in Clancy and Gauthier (eds), *Health Services Research (HSR),* Special Supplement, Part II, 39(4): 1123–1140.

Clancy, C. and A. Gauthier (eds) (2004) "Consumer-directed health care: beyond rhetoric with research and experience," *Health Services Research (HSR),* Special Supplement, Part II, 39(4): 1049–1233.

Davis, K. (2004) "Consumer-directed health care: will it improve health system performance?", in Clancy and Gauthier (eds), *Health Services Research (HSR),* Special Supplement, Part II, 39(4): 1219–1231.

Fowles, J. *et al.* (2004), "Early experience with employee choice of consumer-directed health plans and satisfaction with enrollment," in Clancy and Gauthier (eds), *Health Services Research (HSR),* Special Supplement, Part II, 39(4): 1141–1158.

Gabel, J., H. Whitmore and Sasso Lo (2004), "Employers" contradictory views about consumer-driven health care: results from a national survey," *Health Affairs*—Web exclusive, 25(6): W4210-W4218.

Ginsburg, P. (2007), "Patients can't do it alone," The Commonwealth Fund, New York, www.Commonwealth Fund.org/publications/publications_show.htm?doc_id 520 260.

Goodman, J. (2006), "What is consumer-directed health care?", *Health Affairs*—Web exclusive, 25(6): W540-W543.

Halvorson, G. (2004), "Commentary—current MSA theory: well meaning but futile," in Clancy and Gauthier (eds), *Health Services Research (HSR),* Special Supplement, Part II, 39(4): 1119–1122.

Herzlinger, R. (2007), *Who Killed Health Care?* New York: McGraw-Hill.

Kodner, D. (2003), "Consumer-directed services: lessons and implications for integrated systems of care," *International Journal of Integrated Care,* 3: 1–7.

Medicare Prescription Drug, Improvement, and Modernization Act of 2003, Pub. L. no. 108–173, 117 Stat 2066 (2003). Print.

Miller, T. (2006), "Getting on the soapbox: views of an innovator in consumer-directed care," *Health Affairs*—Web exclusive, 25(6): W549-W551.

Newhouse, J. (1993) *Free for All? Lessons from the Rand Insurance Experiment,* Cambridge, MA: Harvard University Press.

Parente, S. (2004), "Evaluation of the effect of a consumer-driven health plan on medical care expenditures and utilization," in Clancy and Gauthier (eds), *Health Services Research (HSR),* Special Supplement, Part II, 39(4): 1189–1209.

Porter, M. and O. Teisberg (2006), *Redefining Health Care: Creating Value-Based Competition on Choice,* Boston: Harvard Business School Press.

Robinson, J.C. (2001), "The end to asymmetric information," *Journal of Health Politics, Policy and Law,* 26(5): 1045.

Scandlen, G. (2004), "Commentary: how a consumer-driven health care evolves in a dynamic market," in Clancy and Gauthier (eds), *Health Services Research (HSR)*, Special Supplement, Part II, 39(4): 1113–1118.

Shearer, G. (2004) "Commentary—defined contribution health plans: attracting the healthy and well-off," in Clancy and Gauthier (eds), *Health Services Research (HSR)*, Special Supplement, Part II, 39(4): 1156–1166.

# 12

# SOCIETAL ALLOCATION OF RESOURCES FOR
# PATIENTS WITH ESRD

I approach the topic of resource allocation for patients with end-stage renal disease (ESRD) with trepidation and chagrin. The trepidation comes from the difficulty of the topic, one that becomes harder, not easier, as time goes on. More people need dialysis, more can benefit from it, more seem inappropriate users, and more and more money is needed to pay for it. How are we supposed to deal with that? The chagrin comes from the fact that I have been saying for at least 20 years, in a voice reminiscent of Chicken Little, "this can't go on, it just can't." But it has gone on and, in the near term, will no doubt continue to go on.

I am relieved to note that I am not alone in my dire, so far unfulfilled, predictions. Richard Rettig, our most distinguished and perceptive American commentator on ESRD over the years, has said much the same thing: "short-term cost containment pressures will be severe . . . and the longer-term issue of limiting access to care cannot be avoided forever" (Rettig, 1996, p. 1123). Moreover, when the much discussed 1984 book, *Painful Prescription: Rationing Hospital Care*, was published, detailing for an American audience the United Kingdom practice of setting a *de facto* covert age limit for dialysis, it was not hard to imagine something like that eventually happening in the United States as well (Aaron and Schwartz, 1984). Yet it has not happened, as least so far as can be seen. To add further confusion, more recent reports from the United Kingdom indicate that dialysis-rationing is not nearly so severe there any longer, even though the proportion of gross domestic product spent on health care in the United Kingdom has not notably increased over the years—the money must be taken from somewhere else (Nicholson, 1998; Chandna et al., 1999).

I mention these points to underscore what should by now be obvious: there is no rational way to predict how the United States (and maybe other countries as well) will respond to financial stress due to ESRD or to any other medical condition. The United States could conceivably muddle through for the indefinite future, wringing its collective hands now and then, introducing one cost-cutting scheme after another to save the day. Or there could be a future national financial crisis, forcing severe changes—even though some of us will take care not to predict just when that will happen. Another alternative would be to say that, even if we are experiencing no palpable crisis, we ought to be doing so, that it is wasteful and irresponsible to be spending so much money on ESRD when there are far more pressing medical and health care needs.

## THE FUTURE FORESHADOWED

However the country comes out on allocating resources to ESRD in the long run, two preliminary considerations are worth noting. One of them foreshadows the kind of problems that would become endemic if our country ever gets universal health care: every major disease would run the risk of incurring an ever-growing budget if it had cost controls no more effective than the present federal ESRD budget—up, up, and away. The other point is that, at least with dialysis, ESRD is the very model of a problem that is already endemic, that is, a severe, life-threatening disease for which, when dialysis is the only alternative, there is no cure, no inexpensive treatment, and no guarantee that those who receive the available treatment will have a decent quality of life. The AZT "cocktail" for AIDS offers a similar example, as do many forms of desperate chemotherapy for advanced cancer, or efforts to forestall congestive heart failure, or recent drugs to keep Alzheimer's disease at bay for a year or so. The recent history of high-technology innovations is full of examples of expensive treatments producing only marginal benefits—but "marginal" only from some social or financial perspective, but possibly benefiting those who receive them: better marginally treated than wholly dead (if not always).

I begin with these two considerations because it is important to situate the problem of resource allocation for ESRD in the right way. I confess I do not really know just what the "right" way is, but I will offer some considered guesses about where policy might move. A wrong way of going should at once be put aside. That is to deal with it as an *ad hoc* problem, taking it out of the context of the health care system as a whole.

The characteristic way this is done is simply to ask "How much should a country be spending on ESRD?" There is no reasonable way of answering that question without nesting it within a number of far broader questions. There is the economist's classic query about the opportunity costs of the program: are there some other ways of spending the money that would produce a better overall health outcome for the country? To which the answer is: possibly so. There is the egalitarian's question whether it is fair to single out—without any comparative policy analysis at all—one disease among many and make it, and it alone, the beneficiary of a seemingly limitless federal entitlement? To which the answer is simple: no.

Then there is the question that devotees of quality-adjusted life years (QALYs) and disability-adjusted life years (DALYs) can ask, whether there is a good return for the money (Harris, 1987; Barker and Green, 1996; Bleichrodt and Johannesson, 1997; Hyder et al., 1998; Murray and Acharya, 1998)? To which the answer is: well, it is a better investment than, say, bone marrow transplants for late-stage breast cancer, which is widely used despite the lack of any good evidence of its efficacy.

There is, finally, the question an advocate of formal priority setting for limited health care budgets can ask: after a lengthy public debate and a comparison with other health care needs, what priority would ESRD merit (Donaldson and Mooney, 1991; Ham, 1997)? Maybe not as high as at present, which is in effect at the very top of the list—but then it is the only disease as such on the entitlement list in the United States. In any event, most present trends indicate that the future of health care in the United States will be marked by a general increase in medical and economic circumstances similar to those characteristic of ESRD. It thus stands as an apt model of what will increasingly be a generic resource allocation issue.

My approach to the problem will begin with a number of assumptions, none of which I believe are particularly controversial (Levinsky and Rettig, 1991; Nissenson and Rettig, 1999; Rettig, 1996). For the foreseeable future it is reasonable to expect that dialysis will, in the absence of a sufficient supply of transplantable kidneys, be the main line of defense against ESRD; that the number of dialysis patients will continue to grow and that the majority of patients in the future will be over 65, with a potentially great (though not inevitable) increase of those over 75; that the future of the ESRD program will be affected by the future of Medicare's more general response to the costs of care for the elderly; that the cost per patient will continue to climb, fueled by improved technology and greater longevity on dialysis; that the quality of life on dialysis will remain poor, even if acceptable to most of those receiving it; and that, in general, the benefit of dialysis will remain marginal, offering a costly treatment with a comparatively short life expectancy. This last-mentioned feature places it in the growing category of other marginal treatments that do not cure, do not offer a restoration to normal functioning, but expensively prolong a life of chronic invalidism, all of which may be acceptable, if not prized, by patients.

My final assumption, tentatively at least for most of this paper, is the most stark: it will be necessary in the United States in the near future, as Medicare runs into more serious problems, to limit the ESRD program, and that will principally mean limiting dialysis. The sooner there is a national debate about how to do that, the better. The public will not then be surprised by what could appear a precipitate conclusion. Note that I do not assume a solution to the shortage of donated organs or that xenotransplantation will come along to save the day. Sobriety requires that an analysis of resource allocation problems does not assume a great technological breakthrough; that is just a way of evading the problem. If such a breakthrough should come, then well and good, that would be wonderful, but that possibility is no excuse not to use the knowledge and information at hand—and only that—as the foundation for any serious reflection on the allocation problem.

## TACTICS FOR THE CONTROL OF COSTS

There are probably no more than four possible ways of controlling—that is, of limiting—ESRD expenditures in the future, and in one way or another each is a form of rationing: (1) to establish publicly visible and known criteria of a medical kind for treatment eligibility as a federal entitlement; (2) to establish a publicly visible age limit on entitlement; (3) to establish some kind of budget cap on dialysis expenditures but leave the choice of eligible patients up to physician discretion; and (4) to use a means-testing approach.

That none of these approaches has passed muster in the past is no reason not to reconsider them. As long as money was, and still is, available to provide dialysis to all comers, and the day of reckoning always put off, there was no real incentive to ration—and plenty of political and other reasons to dodge the matter altogether. My discussion presupposes *ex hypothesis* that the problem *must* be solved, and that the available choices will each be unpleasant, probably painful. We will then be faced with a classical moral and political problem, that of choosing the least bad solution.

## EXPLICIT, PUBLICLY KNOWN MEDICAL CRITERIA FOR ELIGIBILITY

At first glance, the idea of specifying medical criteria as the basis for an entitlement seems obvious and fair. It is obvious in the sense that it appears compatible with recent efforts to establish evidence-based medicine as a key component of efficient, cost-effective health care: provide treatment when the evidence for its efficacy is, on balance, strong. It seems fair because it does not use any criteria other than impersonal medical benefits as a means of distributing scarce resources. The use of QALYs has been one frequently proposed method for making such determinations, with DALYs as an alternative approach. In both cases, the specific aim of these techniques has not been to determine if a particular patient should receive a treatment but whether a class of treatments (e.g., dialysis) offers a better use of resources than some alternative uses of the same resources (e.g., prenatal screening programs). These techniques could be adapted to screen individual patients.

For all of its apparent moral congeniality (if I may so put it), efforts to specify medical criteria for the treatment of life-threatening conditions have never fared well (save for cardiopulmonary resuscitation with terminally ill patients). The main objection has focused on the discrepancy between what outside observers take to be a life of acceptable quality and functioning and what patients themselves consider tolerable (Evans *et al.*, 1985). It is a common phenomenon (and not just with dialysis) that people adapt to a loss of function and an increase in pain and discomfort much better than they themselves expect in advance. The fashioning of a new self-identify is probably the necessary price to be paid for such adaptation, but it can be and is commonly achieved. The elderly seem more able to change in that respect than the young. If they are no longer working, and no longer have the responsibility for child care, they have the time and possibility of living with conditions that might undo younger people.

Now it might well be argued that, even if patients are prepared to put up with a low quality of life for a short period of time, dialysis is simply not a good investment of societal resources. Surely better ways of spending the money to improve health could be found. With that kind of judgment in mind, it might be perfectly possible to fashion some strict treatment standards. But the almost immediate retort to such a proposal is to ask: but whose standard of the quality of life is to be used? That of some expert body or commission, or the patient's physician, or the consensus of nephrologists? But who can claim to be an "expert" on what kind of life is worth living? Recall the title of a play from the 1970s: *Whose Life Is It Anyway?*. If it is the length of life after a treatment that is at stake, a seemingly objective enough criterion, little imagination is required to think of people who, for family or other reasons, would be happy to have a few more years, just a few; and, in any case, much money is spent in other health domains where the prospects are no better.

Surely it might be possible to fashion some ostensibly "objective" medical standards for eligibility. But it would be hard to demonstrate to almost one and all that they were not arbitrary and that they did not seem to impose some stranger's notion of what would count as a life worth living, or a life worth saving. Anything less than meeting that stringent test would have a poor chance of gaining political acceptance.

## AGE-BASED ELIGIBILITY LIMITS

Since the greatest increase in dialysis patients in recent years has been among those over age 65, with even greater increases expected in the future, it is only reasonable to consider the use of age itself as a standard for the setting of limits (Callahan, 1987). An age limit of, say, 70 or 75 for dialysis eligibility could make an enormous financial difference (and, for the record, I write this as someone who is now 70; hence, it is "us" I am talking about, not "them").

Apart from simply saving money, an age limit would have three advantages. First, it would use an objective standard, chronological age, that could be equitably applied to everyone, much as a driving age of 16, or a drinking age of 21, is applied to the young in the United States—and of course it is a standard, with 65 as the starting point, for the US Medicare program itself. Few have ever claimed that the use of 65, a specific age, as a requirement for Medicare eligibility is itself unfair or ageist, even though many have sought to lower that age to take care of those in need below that line. Second, unless one holds that it is the purpose of medicine, and the goal of federal entitlement programs, to carry out an unrelenting war against death, whatever a person's age and whatever the cost, then there is nothing inherently wrong in allowing someone to die from disease in old age. Few previous cultures have considered such deaths evil (even though they often did consider them sad) (Reynolds, 1991). A reasonable goal for a healthcare system is to help the young become old, not to help old people become indefinitely older.

Third, since it is the working young who pay for most healthcare costs of the elderly, it can be an unfair burden on them to demand that they support an unrelenting battle against mortality in old age, and at that time of life when they have their own families and lives to support. Money taken from the young to pay for the old, particularly if too much money, can also be seen as money that might better be used to improve the health of the young—to help them become old. Nor can it plausibly be argued that, because they will when they become old be the beneficiaries of the next younger generation, there is no problem in their now paying for the present healthcare costs of the elderly. Those costs could, if significantly increased, still be an enormous burden, crippling their ability to meet the present needs of their families. It may be a consolation that they will have a better future when old—but that does not help pay their present bills.

Despite what have always seemed to me some compelling arguments in favor of age-based rationing, I soon discovered it is an idea that just about everyone loves to hate (Barry and Bradley, 1991; Binstock and Post, 1991; Varekamp, 1998). For many it reeks of ageism, that of using chronological age to stigmatize the old, putting them in a category they have no choice about and then using that to deny them life-saving or life-improving treatments. The campaign against age-ism, inspired in great part by the work of Robert Butler in the 1970s, has worked relentlessly to demolish stereotypes about the old and to give them a full share of life unburdened by fixed and often mythical ideas about old age (Butler, 1975). It is then a bucket of harshly cold water to reintroduce age as a standard for discriminatory use, to in effect blame the elderly—so the charge goes—for being a social and economic burden.

A no less common objection is that the aged are an exceedingly heterogeneous group, more so than other age groups, and that a person's chronological age is a meaningless predictor of a person's health or life prospects. An age-based rationing standard would be grossly unjust, treating every elderly person alike, though they are not, and ignoring massive evidence of the gap between chronological age, on the one hand, and health and quality of life, on the other. It could also produce the perverse result of allowing younger people with poor health prospects to receive care that would be denied an older person with otherwise good, even better, health prospects.

## FIXED BUDGETS AND PHYSICIAN DISCRETION

The essence of the United Kingdom way of controlling the cost of dialysis is by forcing doctors to live with fixed budgets but at the same time allowing them considerable freedom in deciding how to spend the money they are allotted. The high cost of dialysis and its obviously heavy burden on any fixed budget makes it a natural target for rationing, particularly for the elderly. (Wing, 1990). The rationing in the United Kingdom is accomplished not by any formal, explicit rules against dialysis for the old, but by informally limiting referrals to specialist consultants who treat ESRD. The rationale given to patients is typically not an economic rationale at all, but instead a medical excuse; that is, that a patient is just not a good candidate for dialysis. A medical myth is thus maintained, seemingly having nothing to do with health-care budgets.

While the average age of referrals to dialysis has gone up significantly in recent years, well above the age 55 first reported in *The Painful Prescription*, the dialysis rate in the United Kingdom is still below that of the United States. There is also a great variation in those rates and the informal age standards from region to region. Better informed and more aggressive patients, moreover, know how to use pressure and knowledge to gain dialysis that might otherwise be denied.

In their much praised book *Tragic Choices*, Guido Calabresi and Philip Bobbit (1978) argued that when societies are faced with unpalatable tragic choices they will frequently hide those choices. That is what the British have traditionally done with dialysis, right up to the present, and there is some evidence this happens in Canada as well (Levine, 1998; McKenzie, 1998). The advantages of this strategy are many: it avoids the nasty politics of open rationing, it allows physicians considerable freedom to do as they choose, and it offers patients a plausible reason for the care denied to them. The disadvantages are no less apparent: the public is deceived about what is going on; physicians are given discretionary power but with no formal accountability for its use; and there is no open debate about where, if rationing is needed, it should at best be focused. Dialysis is picked on principally because of its cost.

At the same time, I should note, I have heard many American nephrologists say that they feel their hands are tied by the present system. Since the treatment is provided free by Medicare, there are no economic reasons to say no to patients, and because the patient is left to be the final judge of what constitutes an acceptable reason for going on dialysis, the physician's judgment is bypassed. If United Kingdom physicians are effectively forced by budget restraints to say no to some patients, they are also left with the freedom to use their clinical judgment to say yes. In that sense, they have the best of both worlds: they can provide dialysis if they choose to do so on clinical grounds, and they can use clinical grounds as a cover for an economic decision if they choose not to do so.

But it is precisely this combination of discretion and disingenuousness that can be the source of injustice and an arbitrary use of physician power. It is hard to imagine that this kind of system would be acceptable in the United States, though not hard to imagine that something like it might be tried. If dialysis was ever put in the hands of health maintenance organization managers who had to live with tight budgets, subterfuge of this kind might well be tempting (though I would hope that the temptation would be rejected and more open, fairer methods of rationing chosen).

### Means-testing

As has been much discussed in the debate about the future of Medicare, the idea of some form of means-testing offers one seemingly attractive option. The argument is simple and straightforward: why should patients receive free what they could afford to pay for, in whole or part? This argument applies, for example, in the United States where the Medicare program as a whole is projected to run into devastating financial problems in the years ahead (Bipartisan Commission, 1994). Even if some strict means-testing plan seems unfeasible—cutting the highly affluent off from the entitlement altogether—would it not at least make sense to institute some kind of co-payment plan, scaling it according to ability to pay? To add strength to such arguments, public opinion surveys in the United States have shown that some form of means-testing is, at this point, about the only acceptable way of controlling Medicare costs (Kaiser Family Foundation/Harvard School of Public Health, 1998).

Yet neither the commonsensical quality of the arguments nor the findings of public opinion polls will necessarily carry the day. In the United States, a large number of people believe that Medicare is an entitlement program that is not an act of charity by Congress, but something that people are owed by virtue of money taken from them by payroll taxes over the years. It is an entitlement based on a congressional promise to return benefits based on worker's contributions over the years. Many liberals look with horror at the idea of means-testing, not so much because the affluent would have to pay for what is now free, but because Medicare has always been seen as a forerunner of universal health care and a model of the way the health care system as a whole should be run.

There are some even more severe economic concerns about means-testing, at least if it is seen as a cost-saving panacea. The high average cost of dialysis, now over $50,000 a year, would put it either totally out of the range of most elderly people or force many of them to beggar themselves to find the money (as is often now the case with long-term care). Some people could surely pay for it, but probably not enough—and especially those over 75—to realize significant savings. The fact that minorities, and African-Americans in particular, are far more likely than whites to suffer from ESRD and are also poorer in old age, would almost surely raise the specter of racism if means-testing was required; and that would be true, I suspect, even if few blacks would be kept from dialysis because of such tests.

As for younger people, now covered by Medicare for ESRD, if they ended in the marginal category of those too well-off to qualify for full coverage but not well-off enough to comfortably afford the costs of a frugal means-testing program, many would be faced with giving up a large portion of their income needed for their own families. The history of Medicare offers many cautionary tales about means-testing, from fraud in gaining coverage, through the indignity of financial screening, to the point of just missing the eligibility cut-off point. The fact that the large majority of the 44 million or so uninsured in the United States have too high an income to qualify for Medicaid, but not enough money to afford health insurance, is not a history encouraging to the idea of means-testing.

## NO EXIT?

A review of the history of arguments about controlling the escalating costs of the ESRD program, and of US Medicare more generally, is not one to encourage optimism about setting limits for that program. Just about every possible policy direction has its critics lined up and ready to leap out with their knives sharpened. But haven't I forgotten one possible policy solution? What about having a fixed or otherwise limited budget and then organizing local or regional committees to make patient-by-patient allocation decisions? If that idea sounds familiar, it is because that is where the dialysis struggle first began in the early 1970s when dialysis machines were in short supply.

As is well known and often recalled, a committee in Seattle was formed to choose patients for the limited number of machines. It turned out to be terrible to make such decisions, to pit one life against another, and it was the failure of that committee to find a satisfactory way of making its decisions that was responsible in part for the 1972 ESRD legislation. One might speculate, moreover, whether it would not now be even more difficult to cut back on a long-standing entitlement, forged out of distress at the prospect of nasty rationing, when it was to put it into place at the outset. My guess is that it would be, but much will depend on available resources.

Another reflection suggests itself when the history of ESRD legislation in the United States is considered. The failure of Congress to create comparable entitlement programs for other diseases—or the universal health care necessary to cover all diseases—suggests that it learned a kind of lingering, hard-to-forget lesson: once open-ended entitlement programs are in place, it will be exceedingly difficult to reduce their coverage if life itself is at stake. The mid-1970s was one of those periods when talk of universal health care was once again in the air in the United States, and a bipartisan bill toward that end was introduced—unsuccessfully—in the US Senate by Senators Edward M. Kennedy and Jacob Javits in 1975. At least one reason it failed was precisely an anxiety about the control of costs once such a program was underway. The Medicare program, and the ESRD program, both of which saw costs quickly escalating beyond early predictions, were object lessons hard to ignore.

Is there no exit here? The picture I have drawn is one in which every way out seems blocked by ethical and political objections, and they have been sufficient to keep the ESRD program going. I say "sufficient" because it is likely also the case that there has always been enough money available from the US federal government to pay for the program, and that has been the "necessary" condition for its continuance.

There are three plausible future possibilities, each of them stemming from quite different situations but all pointing to the same policy outcome. One of them is a severe national economic crisis at some point in the future, an epic depression, forcing cutbacks in even the most well-established and popular entitlement programs. Another is the prospect of severe rationing in the next 20 years or so as the Medicare program (and perhaps other national health programs) is forced to reduce its pace of program growth needed to keep up with the retiring baby boom generation. Still another prospect is that, finally, a universal health care bill will be passed. If that is the case, and if the cost of such a bill is to be sustainable, then there will have to be some rationing (as is the case in every other country with such legislation).

Whichever of these possibilities presents itself, something would have to be done about the program. And at that point, the strategies I discussed above—all of which have hitherto been found wanting—would have to be reconsidered. I have long felt that, for the reasons outlined above, a formal age limit on expensive, high-technology medicine (though coupled with good primary care as well as decent long-term care) would be the fairest solution—if democratically implemented, and with the agreement of the elderly themselves. But no country has ever put in place such a formal policy and I have come to doubt that any country, and particularly the United States, ever will. Politically, it would be much too blunt and much too easy to identify those who would be the losers under such a policy.

Indeed, if the past history of efforts to ration health care is any guide, no policy that is too open in its tactics and whose victims would be too easily identifiable is likely to succeed politically. The rationing would have to be obscured by ambiguous policies and its victims be "statistical" not identifiable victims. That would also mean that the use of specific medical criteria for denying treatment would have to be ruled out as well. For it too would have identifiable victims. I say this not out of cynicism but because it is probably true, as Calabresi and Bobbit (1978) argued in *Tragic Choices*, that it is too hard to openly face truly nasty decisions. An official pretense of ignorance at what is happening will most likely prevail.

If that last speculation is correct, that leaves two realistic possibilities. Means-testing is one of them, almost certain in any case for the future of Medicare in the United States, and likely to gain public support. But, as suggested earlier, that policy would probably not realize a significant saving, given the high annual cost of dialysis and the likelihood that the majority of patients could not afford it.

We are left then with the plausible possibility of forcing physicians to work with set budgets, leaving it to them to make the hard decisions behind a veil of discretion if not secrecy—but sparing them, in return, from invasive oversight and the threat of law suits and criminal prosecution. That is the way the United Kingdom system has been run, and not unsatisfactorily even though there are from time to time complaints about the denial of life-saving treatments to patients. But these complaints have not been effective in increasing the budget of the National Health Service. There are, as noted, great possibilities for injustice to individuals in that kind of system, but also tacit respect for the needs of different age groups. An open-ended spending of money to extend the life of the elderly, who have already run the race of life, is not considered a "need" of the elderly as a group.

There is one option I have not explored here, and to me it would be the ideal. It would be a priority-setting scheme along the lines of that now used by the US state of Oregon in its Medicaid program for the poor. That scheme blends public contributions and professional judgment, to develop a rank-ordering of treatments, to be funded according to the available budget allocated by legislatures. But no other state has chosen to emulate Oregon, and it is even less likely it could be achieved at a national level. In the Oregon plan, moreover, life-saving therapies have a high ranking and it is easily imaginable that they would continue to do so in any other state or national plan (because of the identifiable victim stigma).

There is one final plausible possibility, flying in the face of my initial assumption that something decisive must be done about the ESRD program: that the United States will remain prosperous enough, and the critics of rationing strong enough, that muddling through as is now done will continue to prevail. There would surely be much nibbling around the edge of the program, shaving costs, cutting moral corners—continuing to refuse, for instance, to build inflation into dialysis reimbursement as is now the case—and maybe some discreet *ad hoc* rationing at the bedside by physicians, but leaving an intact if increasingly starved program.

The United States has proven itself exceedingly adept at not solving, or even directly confronting, long-standing problems. That one generation of reformers after another ever since the Second World War has predicted, wrongly so far, the creation of a universal health plan tells a sad but persistent story of hopes dashed and irrationality continued. The ESRD story may, for some at any rate, have a somewhat different and happier moral. That is the capacity of the country to continue financing a program that has so much going against it financially, and yet has saved so many lives over the years. For those who hold this view, it will be the capacity of the ESRD program to *resist* radical reform that will be the great victory.

*References*

Aaron, H. J., and Schwartz, W. B. (1984). *Painful prescription: Rationing hospital care.* The Brookings Institution, Washington.

Barker, C, and Green, A. (1996). Opening the debate on QALYs. *Health Policy and Planning,* 11,179–83.

Barry, R. L., and Bradley, G. V. (1991). *Set no limits: A rebuttal to Daniel Callahan's proposal to limit health care for the elderly.* University of Illinois Press, Urbana, IL.

Binstock, R. H., and Post, S. G. (1991). *Too old for health care?* The Johns Hopkins University Press, Baltimore, MD.

Bipartisan Commission on Entitlement and Tax Reform (1994). *Final Report.* Superintendent of Documents, Washington.

Bleichrodt, H., and Johannesson, M. (1997). The Validity of QALYs. *Medical Decision Making,* 17,21–32.

Butler, R. N. (1975). *Why survive? Being old in America.* Harper & Row, New York.

Calabresi, G., and Bobbit, P. (1978). *Tragic choices.* W. W. Norton, New York.

Callahan, D. (1987). *Setting limits: Medical goals in an aging society.* Simon & Schuster, New York.

Chandna, J. M., Schulz, J., Lawrence, C, Greenwood, R. N., and Farrington, K., (1999). Is there a rationale for rationing chronic dialysis? *British Medical Journal,* 318, 217–223.

Donaldson, C., and Mooney, M. (1991). Needs assessment, priority setting, and contracts for health care: An economic view. *British Medical Journal,* 303, 1529–1530.

Evans, R. W., *et al.* (1985). The quality of life of patients with end-stage renal disease. *The New England Journal of Medicine,* 312, 553–559.

Ham, C. (1997). Priority setting in health care: Learning from international experience. *Health Policy,* 42, 49–66.

Harris, J. (1987). QALYfying the value of life. *Journal of Medical Ethics,* 13, 117–123.

Hyder, A. A., Rotllant, G., and Morrow, R. H. (1998). Measuring the Burden of Disease: Healthy Life Years. *American Journal of Public Health,* 88, 196–202.

Kaiser Family Foundation/Harvard School of Public Health (1998). *National survey on Medicare: The next big health policy debate?* The Kaiser Family Foundation, Menlo Park, California.

Levine, D. Z. (1998) Would you deny this patient dialysis? *American Journal of Diseases,* 31, 131–132.

Levinsky, N. G., and Rettig, R. A. (1991). The Medicare end-stage renal disease program. *The New England Journal of Medicine,* 324,1143–1148.

McKenzie, J. K. (1998) Dialysis decision making in Canada, the United Kingdom, and the United States. *American Journal of Kidney Diseases,* 31,12–18.

Murray, C. J. L., and Acharya, A. K. (1997). Understanding DALYs. *Journal of Health Economics,* 16,703–730.

Nicholson, R. H. (1998). Truth lies somewhere if we knew but where. *Hastings Center Report,* 22,1999.

Nissenson, A. R., and Rettig, R. A. (1999). Medicare's end-stage renal disease program: current status and future prospects. *Health Affairs,* 18,161–179.

Rettig, R. A. (1996). The social contract and the treatment of permanent kidney failure. *Journal of the American Medical Association,* 275,1123–1126.

Reynolds, R. (1991). Natural death: A history of religious perspectives. In *Life span: Values and life-extending technologies* (ed. Veatch, R. M.). Harper & Row, New York, 145–161.

Varekamp, L. J. (1998). Age rationing for renal transplantation? The role of age in decisions regarding scarce life extending medical resources. *Social Science and Medicine,*
47,113–120.

Wing, A. J. (1990). Can we meet the real need for dialysis and transplantation? *British
Medical Journal,* 301, 897–890.

# 13

# SHAPING BIOMEDICAL RESEARCH PRIORITIES: THE CASE OF THE NATIONAL INSTITUTES OF HEALTH

At least in theory, if hardly yet in adequate practice, the movement to establish the value of priority setting for health care seems by now to be well advanced. It is marked by a number of national commissions, an international organization, and a variety of efforts to devise appropriate priority setting mechanisms (Ham, 1997). But there is also a striking anomaly in that movement: with a few exceptions, priority setting for biomedical research has been altogether neglected (Commission on Health Research, 1990; Report of the Ad Hoc Committee, 1996). The emphasis has instead been on the allocation and delivery of health care services.

While that latter emphasis has surely been understandable—a function of the economic and other pressures experienced by national health care systems—biomedical research no less merits attention. That research will, after all, create most of the new drugs and technologies that future health care systems will be called upon to provide, disseminate—and prioritize. If one can reasonably ask how present health care can more fairly and efficiently be distributed, and with what priorities, it is no less reasonable to ask just what kind of future health care possibilities we might like to see research make available.

I will not attempt here to lay out a full theory of priority setting for biomedical research—something still marinating in my mind—but just present what I take to be important considerations in such an effort. After attempting to distinguish between priority setting for health care delivery and for biomedical research, I will move on to the current debate about priority setting at the National Institutes of Health (NIH) in Washington. It provides a most useful and timely case study. With the salient details of that debate in place, I will draw some conclusions about what a more robust and systematic process of research priority setting might look like.

## SIMILARITIES AND DIFFERENCES

There are some obvious similarities between health care priority setting and research priority setting. Both have been motivated by the clamor of various constituencies asking for increased resources or complaining that they have not received a fair share of the available resources. Both have been prodded by a perceived need for a way of allocating scarce resources that is more rational and equitable. Both have sought methods of priority setting that will simultaneously satisfy health care professionals and the general public.

If those are some of the important similarities, two points need to be made at once. The first is that the effort to devise priorities for health care systems is far more advanced and sophisticated than for biomedical research. With the exception of the NIH, it is hard to discover much extended debate anywhere in the world on how best to prioritize research, though examples now and then emerge. The second point is that, while there are many similarities in the efforts of each, there are some important differences. On the whole, I have come to think, while it is hard enough to devise a good methodology for health care priority setting— not to mention getting governments to actually adopt one scheme or another—it is even harder to do so for biomedical research. A look at some of the differences between the two will help underscore that point.

The aim of setting priorities for health care delivery is to find a fair and rational way of meeting current health care needs with the resources currently available. The aim of priority setting for biomedical research, also with the available resources, is (a) in the short run to improve medical knowledge and the tools necessary to meet current and near-future health care needs, and to ameliorate or cure those diseases and maladies that create such needs; and (b) in the long run to gain a better understanding of the underlying biological processes responsible for disease and disability in order to find cures and/or decisively effective therapies with which to treat them.

Biomedical research has characteristically been classified as basic and applied. The former typically refers to the gaining of new and fundamental biological knowledge, the utility of which for improving health may at the moment of discovery be unknown or even non-existent. The latter refers to targeted research, ordinarily aimed at the cure or treatment of a specific medical condition. Now while it has become increasingly popular to deny that, in practice, there is any significant difference between basic and applied research (each can supply insights into the other in unpredictable ways), there can be little doubt that the difference is meaningful to scientists. It is the difference between wanting to know something for its own sake—simply how the biological world is constructed—and wanting to know something for the sake of improving health. To be sure, both of those aims can be sought at the same time, but it is still useful to distinguish logically between them because they have different implications for priority setting, as the NIH debate (to which I will shortly come) makes clear.

For the moment, it is important simply to note that while priority setting for health care delivery is concerned only with meeting present needs, research aims at future as well as present needs. It also aims, more radically, at gaining the kind of deeper basic biological knowledge that will enable future generations to deal with new and changing health and disease conditions as they emerge. It is not, then, that research is disinterested in current health problems. Not at all. In fact, it is those problems that typically command the greatest research resources (at least at NIH). But it is also the case that research seeks *more* than simply meeting present needs, which is why it is important to note the visionary thrust of basic research (and of that applied research which may throw off unexpected knowledge of long-term value). Unlike allocating resources to the provision of health care, where the likely benefits can be fairly predictable, biomedical research is much less certain in its outcome. The usual bet is that, even if exact benefits cannot be predicted, some benefits can be expected, particularly if negative results are counted a gain, as is common among researchers.

## THE CASE OF NIH

I have discussed the aims of research not simply to make some necessary distinctions, but also because the debates over the years at NIH have turned, in great part, on the goals and purposes of that institution. Formed just prior to World War II, the NIH grew rapidly after the War. Its growth was stimulated by the medical progress made during the War; by the great push given to all scientific research in the postwar years; by considerable public support for biomedicine; and by the promise of great strides against the killer diseases, especially cancer. From the outset there was a struggle between an important segment of the scientific community that looked to NIH to provide funds for basic research, carried out at the initiative of the scientists themselves, and other scientists with considerable lay support who pressed for targeted, applied research (Strickland, 1972; Spingarn, 1976).

The former group of scientists was hardly uninterested in improving health or gaining the kind of biological knowledge that could be turned to useful clinical practice. But they believed that the free and unimpeded pursuit of basic scientific knowledge was the best way to get there. Again and again, they liked to note, some of the most important knowledge in the struggle against disease has come from serendipity, unexpected benefits from research with no specific clinical purposes in mind.

But the scientific voice was not the only important voice, nor were all of the scientists of one mind. Hardly less important as time went on was the influence of some vigorous disease-advocacy groups, intent that their disease receive earmarked funds, and of some members of Congress, who felt that a large allocation of funds to the NIH required practical and visible results, most notably an improvement in health and progress against disease and disability. The lay advocates of targeted research, with the support of like-minded scientists, were particularly effective in their lobbying activities. Taken together, they were a powerful force in gaining a steady increase in NIH funding (Strickland, 1978).

To its credit, the Congress over the decades managed to listen sympathetically to both groups and to achieve a good balance of interests. While it has frequently heeded the lobbyists—mandating new programs and centers, and increasing some budgets beyond what NIH has requested—it has also been generous in its support of investigator-initiated research and in giving considerable leeway to the various NIH institutes in setting their own priorities. Neither one side nor the other has ever gained a decisive upper hand, perhaps because both of the general contending positions have maintained at least public respect for the other side.

Of late, however, two events have taken place which add a new chapter to the story. One of them has been a powerful congressional push—not initiated by the NIH—to strikingly increase NIH's annual budget, aiming to double it over the next five years (from $13 billion in 1998 to $26 billion by 2003). This development, with full bipartisan support, bespeaks the high status not only of that agency but of biomedical research as well.

The other event, unfolding over the past few years, has been pressure on NIH to explain and justify its methods for setting priorities. The pressure has come from various disease advocacy groups, claiming their particular disease is not getting a fair share, and from Congress, which has not only listened to those pleas and complaints, but has had some questions of its own (Subcommittee on

Public Health and Safety, 1997). The disease advocacy groups have, in particular, made much of the discrepancy among the various diseases in the amount of research money spent on one disease versus another. HIV/AIDS, for instance, gets $1069 per afflicted patient, while heart disease gets only $93 per patient, and Parkinson's disease still less, at $26 per afflicted patient (Marshall, 1997). The congressional pressure has not been harsh, but it has been persistent, particularly as the NIH budget has grown. At least some observers believe that the recent large increases in the NIH budget, which should please NIH, will be matched by an increase in pressure to justify the way it allocates its funds, which may be less pleasing.

## SETTING PRIORITIES AT THE NIH

In response to the various pressures to explain itself better, the NIH in 1997 issued a white paper "Setting Research Priorities at the National Institutes of Health" (Committee on the NIH Priority-Setting Process, 1998). That paper set forth the complexity of the NIH mission, criteria used to set priorities, the process used in deploying the criteria, and a response to various proposals to use a more objective burden of illness standard in setting priorities.

The complexity of its mission, the paper noted, stems from its aim to simultaneously carry out basic research—which can cut across a number of its institutes and which will often lead to unexpected practical results in the treatment of various diseases—and to do research on specific diseases. But even the latter kind of research is not confined to a specific institute. Accordingly, the paper contends, "There is, consequently, no 'right' amount of money, percentage of the budget, or number of projects for any one disease" (Committee on the NIH Priority-Setting Process, 1998). At the same time, the NIH also has the obligation to provide infrastructure support to the entire biomedical research enterprise in the United States.

## THE CRITERIA USED TO SET PRIORITIES ARE:[1]

—public health needs
—scientific quality of the research
—potential for scientific progress
—portfolio diversification across the broad and expanding frontiers of
  research

—adequate support of infrastructure (human capital, equipment and instrumentation, and facilities).

The process for deploying these criteria is mixed. Congress from time to time mandates particular lines of research, leaving NIH less room to fully use its own criteria. Internally, each institute sets its own priorities using (presumably) these criteria; and the director of the NIH uses them as well, taking into account lay opinion, scientific advice, and internal discussion. While the white paper does describe the process of decision-making in a general way, it is not clear just how formal and systematic it actually is, particularly when the final decisions are made.

Of particular interest is the way the white paper responds to proposals over the years to use some form of a burden of illness standard to set priorities. It notes that the NIH could distribute research funds based on:

—the number of people who have a disease
—the number of deaths caused by a disease
—the degree of disability produced by a disease
—the degree to which a disease cuts short a normal, productive, comfortable lifetime
—the economic and social costs of a disease
—the need to act rapidly to control the spread of a disease

While it does not explicitly say so, any observer familiar with the international priority setting literature can find in that list echoes of the debates about QALYs, DALYs, and HeaLYs. Americans will promptly recall the arguments about funding AIDS and cancer research; squabbles about the recent increases in the budget for Parkinson's disease and diabetes; and complaints that diseases that bring severe disability but not death (such as arthritis) can get short-changed in the competition for funds.

The NIH white paper decisively rejects the use of any one of those possible standards as the sole determinant for priority setting. To use the number of people affected by a disease as the standard could come to emphasize less serious medical conditions (such as the common cold) and have a limited impact on population health. To focus on number of deaths would neglect non-lethal chronic disease and disability and their high societal costs. Yet to focus exclusively on disability or economic costs would raise difficult questions about the feasibility of quantifying them and of calculating both direct and indirect costs. To use economic costs as a sole standard would neglect short illnesses and rapid death (e.g., sudden infant death syndrome). To base funding solely on immediate dangers to public health could take funds away from areas of greater long-term impact.

## PROBLEMS WITH THE NIH METHOD OF PRIORITY SETTING

The NIH method of priority setting might be classified as one using unranked criteria as its principal guidelines and partially informal means of actually using those criteria as its main way of deploying them. That approach can be contrasted with the use in some countries of ranked criteria in a health policy context—such as the priority given to acute and lethal conditions in Norway and Sweden, followed by a ranking of other conditions—and the use of a formal decision-making commission to set numerically ranked criteria, as in Oregon.

The drawbacks of the NIH use of unranked criteria are not hard to discern. There is no suggestion about whether one of the criterion is more important than any other. Is public health really no more important than infrastructure support? There is no hint of how conflicts among the criteria are to be adjudicated. What if the greatest scientific opportunities lie in combating the common cold? The criteria themselves are, moreover, radically dissimilar, lending themselves to no clear means of comparison. How is a balance to be struck between the need of institutions for new equipment and the possibility of progress in understanding Alzheimer' disease? The white paper simply does not address problems of that kind.

To make matters worse, the deployment of those criteria, described in a vague way only—and heavily dependent in the end on decisions taken by NIH leadership—provides no clues about how such conflicts and dilemmas are handled. The NIH argument that no single standard—economic or medical—should be used to set priorities does not confront the obvious point that two or three or more of the standards it rejected if used alone could be combined in some meaningful way. The hinted implication (but only that) of the white paper that they are in fact combined in some fashion—though just how is left opaque—is less than illuminating.

It is hard to avoid an unsettling conclusion: despite what NIH says, theirs is really not quite a priority setting procedure at all. Webster's dictionary defines a priority as "a preferential rating," a definition consistent with other dictionaries, all of which stress ranking as their common element. The lack of a preferential rating or ranking of the criteria it employs, and (at least as viewed from the outside) a reasonably clear process for working with them, deprives its system of the minimal elements necessary to set priorities in a systematic fashion. It may be a method of decision-making, or a method of "this-is-what-we-think-about-as-we-make-our-choice-of-research-allocation-possibilities," but it is not a priority setting *method*, lacking the necessary ingredients to make it so. Without ranking, there are no priorities. To say this is not to deny that, when the final decisions are made, some things will get more money than others, and thus that de facto priorities will be observable. It is only to say that the NIH does not have a priority-setting method in the strict sense of the term.

The NIH method of setting priorities has not gone unchallenged. The Congress was sufficiently concerned to ask the Institute of Medicine (IOM) of the National Academy of Sciences to conduct a study of the way the NIH set priorities. Chaired by a leading and thoughtful scientist and former Dean of the Yale Medical School, Dr. Leon Rosenberg, and working with a tight deadline in the first half of 1998, the committee interviewed key NIH staff members, invited comments from various disease advocacy groups, and sought the judgment of many scientists and their professional organization (Committee on the NIH Research Priority-Setting Process, 1998).

While the IOM committee had a number of recommendations to make, two were of special importance. One of them was that the NIH should have better procedures in place to allow the public to make its views known, and specifically known within the Director's office (by establishing an Office of Public Liaison), a recommendation immediately seized upon (Agnew, 1998; Dresser, 1999). The other was that the NIH should work more diligently to gain knowledge about the burden of illness within the United States, believing that NIH need a better data base for its priority decisions. Additionally the IOM committee recommended greater clarity on the part of NIH in implementing its priorities.

## IF IT AIN'T BROKE, DON'T FIX IT

What stands out in the IOM report is that it expressed no basic dissatisfaction with the way the IOM sets its priorities. In a vein of "if it ain't broke, don't fix it," the report's very first "recommendation" is a broad endorsement of the NIH procedures: "The committee generally supports the criteria that NIH uses for priority setting and recommends that NIH continue to use these criteria in a balanced way to cover the full spectrum of research related to human health."

Since the mere existence of unranked criteria offers no guidance on what counts as a "balanced way" of setting priorities, the committee in effect overlooked or sidestepped the theoretical difficulties of working with non-preferential, unranked criteria. Nor did it make clear just how a greater public input would be used for hard decision-making (many scientists claim there is more than enough already) or what difference better and more extensive burden of illness data would make either. That has not been a Congressional demand and it is by no means certain that Congress would want different priorities even if it had such information. Such information might, however, add some useful information to the budget debates, at least serving as a corrective to poorly based claims and complaints.

In light of the serious substantive problems that can readily be unearthed in the NIH priority setting criteria and processes, what is one to make of the IOM report? One facile answer is that the IOM committee would have profited from a close examination of the international priority setting literature even though it is mainly focused on health care delivery. That would at least have made evident some of the more subtle problems of sophisticated priority setting.

A more pertinent answer is probably that the committee composition (heavily weighted with scientists) and its report reflected a broad and deep consensus within the American biomedical research and clinical community. It is that the NIH is a vital, effective, and well run organization and blessed at the moment with a particularly distinguished and effective leader in Dr. Harold Varmus. Even if, by some more rigorous standards, the IOM report did not go very deeply into priority setting, it was in effect saying: we like what it is doing, we trust its leadership to make good priority decisions, and we see no good reason to shake the faith of the Congress or the general public about the way NIH goes about carrying out its mission.

Now if that interpretation is correct, it surely raises an additional question. If in the end it is a basic trust in NIH and its leadership that is allowed to be the final judge of the way it sets priorities, what would happen with bad leadership? Isn't one point of having a well-defined, organized scheme for setting priorities to allow an institution (or health care system, as the case may be) not only to judge the ways resources are allocated by some higher standards, but also to control the way administrators and others in power actually do so?

Of course that has always been the attraction of some formal, scientifically grounded, putatively objective way of setting priorities. That is why the economic techniques of QALYs, DALYs, and the like have attracted at least academic attention (and a bit more than that in the case of DALYs, officially embraced by the World Bank). And it is surely why another, less noticed, critique of the NIH procedures placed its emphasis almost entirely upon burden of illness studies as the way NIH should set its priorities (and giving the health of the public a clearly higher priority than other NIH goals) (Tengs, 1998).

## SCIENCE, POLITICS AND RATIONALITY

Often enough, I have noticed, the economic and other formal methods of priority setting are called "rational," the implication being that any other method is less than rational or irrational. But the IOM committee—the evidence of the report suggests—tacitly adopted a different standard in making its assessment, one that might be called political and pragmatic. It judged the past and present results of the work of NIH as important and exemplary, however it managed to achieve those goods. It concluded that its leadership is responsible and sensible and that it can work perfectly well with somewhat vague and potentially contradictory priority setting criteria. It almost surely made the political judgment that little good for the future of NIH would come by holding it up to some supposedly higher, more theoretical standard of methodological rationality.

That can be a perfectly sound kind of conclusion. It also suggests to me why politicians and administrators are far less drawn to the more elaborate kinds of priority setting than their advocates might expect and hope for: they are more trustful of politics and pragmatic common sense to deal with the complexity of priority setting than they are of more formal schemes. It is probably no accident that Oregon is the only state to have adopted an explicit priority setting formula. It does not seem to attract legislators. Nor is it probably mere chance that most of the countries that have put together commissions to propose better means of setting priorities have not succeeded in getting their legislators or health care administrators to share their enthusiasm.

For all of its faults, inequities, and irrationalities, what I have called the political method of setting priorities still seems more attractive. It is familiar, messy, and yet comparatively simple in its operation: people argue, struggle, and lobby to get what they want, and there are winners and losers—but also another chance on another day for the losers to turn the tables. By contrast, the more technically sophisticated a priority-setting scheme, the more difficult it is likely to be in gaining support for actual implementation. Burden of illness studies, for all of their elegant attractiveness, are almost always mired in technical disputes among competing experts, but also difficult to carry out even if a consensus on methodology can be reached.

I do not want what I am saying here to be construed as an argument against the search for good methods of setting priorities. I was an early and enthusiastic supporter of the Oregon Medicaid effort to set priorities and of the broader international effort now underway to develop good strategies and methods for priority setting. And better ideas for setting research priorities are in particular short supply. Nonetheless, if the general movement is to get anywhere in the long run, it will be necessary to accomplish two aims. The most evident is the need for good, and politically persuasive, ideas about how best to set priorities, in terms of both substance and process. The less explored, but to my mind no less important, need is to better understand the political and administrative attractiveness of the kind of informal model used at the NIH. It reflects, I am convinced, a way of working with priorities and difficult decisions that is attractive not only in the United States, but in other countries as well.

The Congress wanted to know how NIH sets its priorities, but it did not ask for, nor does it seem to expect, anything too precise or too scientific; and the IOM committee did not look for, much less demand, that either. The IOM report recommended some modest changes perfectly consistent with what NIH is already doing (and some NIH defenders have said "but we're already doing that!" and, to some extent, that is true).

Sympathetic though I am to the political mode of priority setting, in the long run the NIH needs to develop more explicit and refined means of setting priorities. It may not always have good leadership or such a sympathetic and permissive Congress. The more money it gets the higher the stakes. Toward that end, I would like to propose two sets of standards for the setting of priorities. Neither of them were clearly asked for by the IOM report, but they would seem necessary for a long-term improvement in the ways needed to judge the validity and rigor of an institution's way of setting priorities. While I am particularly interested here in research priority setting, they might work equally well with health care delivery. The first set of standards bears on the setting of long-range national health goals—what are we looking for in the long run? The second set are some criteria for evaluating any chosen process of setting priorities.

## NATIONAL HEALTH GOALS

It is, to my mind at least, a curiosity that the National Institutes of Health has set for itself no finite goals. It operates with what one commentator on the idea of progress has called an "unconstrained vision" (Sowell, 1987). By that is meant, in this context, progress without end in the improvement of health. What would count as success in the struggle for good health? That has never been made clear, but presumably (if the implicit logic of the enterprise is examined) nothing less than a full understanding of the origins of diseases and their total eradication would suffice (Callahan, 1998).

To be sure, there are many who find no trouble with such an open-ended agenda, any more than most of us find no trouble with an open-ended program for the exploration of outer space—a space without end. But the NIH would be better served by specifying some discrete and potentially attainable goals. That would help to measure the progress it is making in its support of research and allow a better assessment of what the public is getting for its money. It would no less help to provide a partial antidote to one of the American neuroses affecting the pursuit of the health of the public: the better the health is the worse off we seem to feel and the more health care we demand (Barsky, 1988).

## IWILL SUGGEST SOME GOALS THAT WOULD LEND THEMSELVES TO SUCH AN ANTIDOTE:

—avoidance of premature death (not of death itself), to the extent that most people will live to old age

—reduction of disability, physical and mental, to the degree that it ceases to be a significant social and economic burden

—relief of pain, suffering, and disability to the level that the majority of those liable to suffer from them are able to function effectively as persons, citizens, and workers

—compression of morbidity and successful aging

—the pursuit of basic biological knowledge

The one open ended agenda would be the pursuit of basic biological knowledge, for which no finite goals can sensibly be set. The maintenance of a strong infrastructure would admit of finite goals.

I offer these as illustrative suggestions only, which I will not pursue or defend. The setting of such goals should be a political action, drawing fully upon public and professional opinion after serious and extended discussion. There would inevitably be struggles to define the goals and to give them a reasonably circumscribed meaning. What would "majority" mean in my suggested goals, and would that be sufficient? And what would it mean to speak of "most people" reaching old age? Those, and analogous, questions would be matters for public debate.

Some limitations would be important. The goals should not contain language or aspirations too vague to be meaningful, nor should they be perfectionist goals (e.g., that *every* person should live to old age). The former could render the goals empty of meaningful content, while the latter would be impossible to accomplish, or impossibly expensive even to try. My overall point, though, should be clear enough: without some finite, theoretically achievable goals, it will be hard to set research goals that are feasible and affordable. This is not a scheme to reduce NIH budgets. For some time to come, research budgets would have to remain steady or be increased even to achieve those finite goals. It is simply a plea to deal with a question that can be asked of any human enterprise: tell us what the goal is and how we will know when it is achieved. This can be done with medicine and health care systems, and it could be done with research agendas (The Hastings Center,1996).

## EVALUATION CRITERIA

If finite health policy goals will be needed, so too are a set of criteria for judging whether the effort to set and live with priorities is achieving its purpose. Here is my suggestion for such a set. The criteria should be:

- —*effective* (uses a rational and coherent method for setting rank-ordered priorities)
- —*simple* (not requiring an excessively technical means of creating and managing them, and understandable to the public)
- —*transparent* (the way the priorities are set would be readily visible to the public)
- —*reformable* (open to easy adjustment and change)
- —*equitable* (fair in its allocation of resources)
- —*acceptable* (commands broad public assent)

By these standards, the NIH process falls short. It does not have an *effective* and coherent method for "preferential rating" (to return to the dictionary definition of a priority). It is *simple* enough perhaps, but hardly *transparent*, depending as it ultimately does on decisions not open to public inspection. It is not readily *reformable* (for reasons too complex to go into here) in that early decisions and traditions considerably limit the discretion of NIH in using the money made available to it. Whether it is *equitable* or not is surely open to dispute, but by its lack of meeting the other criteria, it surely opens itself to that charge (though I happen to think it is equitable).

Is the NIH process *acceptable* by the norms I specified? The answer seems to be, against the odds perhaps, *yes*. At the least it is acceptable to Congress, which may mutter but does not revolt; acceptable enough to the scientific community, even if it might do some tinkering; and acceptable to the general public in that the public does not complain about what NIH does nor does it put pressure on Congress to reform the present pattern.

So, when we come to the bottom line, the NIH does exceedingly well. This tells me two things. One of them is that neither the Congress nor the public is longing for greater "rationality," in the way that term is often used by those who have some elegant technical ways of setting priorities waiting in the wings, ready to step on stage if give a chance. The other thing is that, as described above, an imprecise, often messy, perhaps unfair, and surely at times opaque political process is acceptable enough to almost everyone if the result is a good one. By that test, the NIH is triumphant. It is a highly respected organization, the beneficiary of unasked-for budget increases of a striking magnitude, and exceedingly good at what it does.

That constellation of results is hardly an argument against having better means of establishing criteria—and in NIH's case actually having some priorities, a "preferential rating"—but it surely indicates how hard it would be to motivate anything significantly different from what now goes on. My guess in that respect suggests a broader conclusion about the worldwide priority setting movement. It will probably not flourish where there is general satisfaction with the regnant political means of setting (or, usually, not setting) priorities. Put differently, it will almost surely require a widespread unhappiness with the common political methods for something more formal to get off the ground. If this is the case with NIH research priorities, it may well be so in other arenas as well, as suggested by the failure of most governments to adopt recommendations for orderly systems of setting priorities. I happen to believe that priority setting is the wave of the future. At the moment, it is a small ripple yet to develop into a wave.

## Acknowledgement

I wish to acknowledge the support of The Patrick and Catherine Weldon Donaghue Foundation for the research that made this article possible.

## Note

1. I use the list presented in a study carried out by the Institute of Medicine and discussed below because its list was developed from documents and testimony it received, and is thus more precise than that presented in the white paper (Committee on the NIH Research Priority-Setting Process, 1998).

## References

Agnew, B. (1998) NIH Embraces Citizens' Council to Cool Debates on Priorities. *Science* 282, 18–19.

Barsky, A. (1988) *Worried Sick: Our Troubled Quest for Wellness*. Boston: Little, Brown.

Callahan, D. (1998) *False Hopes*. New York: Simon & Schuster.

Commission on Health Research for Development (1990) *Health Research: Essential Link to Equity in Development*. New York: Oxford University Press.

Committee on the NIH Priority-Setting Process (1998) *Scientific Opportunities and Public Need: Improving Priority Setting and Public Input at the National Institutes of Health*. Washington, D.C.: National Academy Press.

Dresser, R. (1999) Public Advocacy and Allocation of Federal Funds for Biomedical Research. *The Milbank Quarterly 77*, 257–274.

Ham, C. (1997) Priority Setting in Health Care: Learning from International Experience. *Health Policy* 42, 49–66.

Marshall, E. (1997) Lobbyists Seek to Reslice NIH's Pie. *Science* 276, 344–346.

NIH Working Group on Priority Setting (1998) *Setting Research Priorities at the National Institutes of Health.* Bethesda: National Institutes of Health (Publication No. 97-4265).

Report of the Ad Hoc Committee on Health Research Relating to Future Interventions (1996) *Investing in Health Research and Development.* Geneva: World Health Organization.

Sowell, T. (1987) *A Conflict of Visions.* New York: William Morrow.

Spingarn, N. (1976) *Heartbeat: The Politics of Health Research.* Washington, D.C.: Robert B. Luce Co.

Strickland, S. (1972) *Politics, Science, and Dread Disease.* Cambridge: Harvard University Press.

Strickland, S. (1978) *Research and the Health of Americans.* Lexington, MA: Lexington Books.

Subcommittee on Public Health and Safety, Committee on Labor and Human Resources, U.S. Senate (1997) *Hearings on Proposed Legislation Authorizing Funds for the National Institutes of Health.* Washington, D.C.: U.S. Government Printing Office.

Tengs, T.O. (1998) *Planning for Serendipity: A New Strategy to Prosper from Health Research.* Washington, D.C.: Progressive Policy Institute.

The Hastings Center (1996). The Goals of Medicine: Setting New Priorities. *Hastings Center Report* 26(Special Supplement), S1–S27.

# 14

# TIME FOR A CHANGE:
# DEVISING OUR MEDICAL FUTURE

For nearly a century, but particularly in the post-WWII era, an unrelenting war against disease has been waged. Richard Nixon's declaration of a war on cancer in 1970 nicely symbolizes that effort. It was matched by a constant and rarely contested increase over the years in the budget of the National Institutes of Health for research on all diseases, a steady rise in life expectancy, numerous health benefits, and an unbounded hope that more and better advances would always be on the way.

Now is the moment to declare a truce in that war. We need to see if the ambitious goals of medical progress still make sense, whether the hope is still justified, and whether an affordable medicine for the future can be fashioned from the values that are now the premises of our health care system.

My answer is no to those goals, hopes, and premises. Not only must the language of war be abandoned but the whole way of thinking that went with it must be put aside, new goals fashioned, and more modest, realistic hopes entertained. The United States saw the financial bubble burst in 2008, a bubble fueled by hype, hope, and reckless spending. The medical bubble is now beginning to burst. Even if the Affordable Care Act (ACA) successfully lets the air out more slowly over the next decade (itself a pious hope), there is no reason to believe costs will permanently stop rising thereafter.

The greatest mistake of the health reform effort has been to assume that finding our way to an economically sustainable future in the face of constantly rising costs is essentially a solvable managerial problem. The evidence suggests otherwise. Every health care system in the developed world—however it is organized—is faced with similar problems: aging societies, expensive technological innovation, and high patient expectations. Utterly missing everywhere in reform debates, but especially in the United States, is a reexamination of some basis assumptions and aspirations of modern medicine. We now have some decades of experience with it, and a reappraisal is in order.

One way to think about those assumptions is to imaginatively cast our mind into the reasonably foreseeable future, say 20 years from now. By then the Baby Boom generation will be at flood tide—rising from 40 million in 2009 to 70 million in 2030—putting enormous pressure on the health care system regardless of how the current reform effort turns out.[1] There is general agreement that the current annual rate of overall system cost escalation, now in the 6%–7% a year range, is intolerable, that it must be brought down to 3% or so, in line with the annual rise in the GDP. What would our system have to look like 20 years from now to make that a plausible goal? My claim is that it is an implausible and unattainable goal without revisiting and shaking up many of the beliefs and values now animating American medicine. There are both philosophical and empirical reasons for doing so.

The guiding premise of our medicine is that the possibilities of medical progress and technological innovation are essentially unlimited, that none of the major lethal diseases is in principle incurable, that more research is the answer to those diseases as well as all the other assorted miseries that can afflict our mind and body, and that the progress is economically affordable if well managed. To constantly fuel this ambitious enterprise, it is necessary to believe in the plausibility of those possibilities, but no less to inspire patients, researchers, and legislators, never to give up hope that they will be achieved. The ancient duty of physicians to instill hope in their sick patients is now matched by the necessity of inspiring ever-refreshed public hope in the medical research enterprise.

Almost every item in the list of major hopes guiding the belief in medical progress should now be questioned. Let me point to some unpleasant realities, beginning with infectious disease. Forty years ago it was commonly assumed that infectious disease had all but been conquered, with the eradication of small pox taken as the great token of that victory. That assumption has been proved false. Infectious disease in the form of epidemic HIV disease, a failure to find cures for malaria and other tropical diseases, and the dangerous increase in antibiotic-resistant microbes make clear that falsity.[2] Not one of those problems is anywhere near a decisive solution. It is only reasonable now to assume that infectious disease will never be eliminated but only, at best, ameliorated. In the absence of a vaccine—despite a nearly 20 years search—the difficulty of keeping up economic support of expensive HIV treatments does not bode well for the ever-increasing number of those who continue to become infected, with steadily growing numbers. One million people live with HIV and AIDS in America, with a fifth of those unaware of their infection.

If costs early on raised their ugly head with HIV disease and its expensive treatment, it is the chronic diseases that are now the scourge of industrialized nations. If the hope for eradication of infectious disease was misplaced, the hope for cures for the leading chronic diseases is no less intoxicated. Richard Nixon's 1970 declaration of a war on cancer, matched by ever-green predictions of an imminent cure, has brought us little closer to that goal. Mortality rates from cancer have only slowly fallen over the decades but the costs of treatment and the prevalence of the disease continue to rise at an alarming rate. A National Cancer Institute study projects a 39% increase in cancer costs between 2010 and 2020.[3] No one of any scientific stature even predicts a cure for heart disease, but expensive ways of keeping those alive with it (especially the elderly) increase. Kidney dialysis is an economic monster, also with a rising number of patients, and with the elderly the largest portion of new patients. A 150% increase in the number of patients is expected over the next decade.[4] As for Alzheimer disease, not long before President Obama announced a fresh effort to find better treatments and a cure, a special panel of the National Institutes of Health determined that essentially little progress has been made in recent years toward finding a cure or even to significantly delay the onset of serious symptoms.[5] The most realistic hopes now lie in the latter category and they are anything but robust. Medicare projects a cost of $91 billion in 2005, growing to $185 in 2015 and $1 trillion in 2050.[6]

Some 64% of health care costs are incurred by 20% of the population with chronic diseases, heavily the elderly. The best that can be said is that medicine has become more and more proficient in keeping sick people, even very sick people, alive longer. Kenneth Thorpe and colleagues, summing up some Medicare data, note that "more than half of all beneficiaries are treated for five or more chronic conditions each year, with 75% making at least one out-patient hospital visit."[7] But that struggle has begun to look like the trench warfare of WWI: little real progress in taking enemy territory but enormous economic and human loses in trying to do so. In that warfare, we can recall, it was the duty of officers to get their soldiers to climb the ramparts and go forth to battle. Medical researchers, industry, and patient advocates play that role in the war against cancer and the other chronic conditions.

One of the hardiest hopes in the chronic disease wars has been that of a compression of morbidity—a long life with little illness followed by a quick death. First developed by James Fries in 1980 it has had the special attraction of a kind of persuasively utopian view of the future of medicine.[8] And it has always been possible to identify very old people who seemed to have the good fortune of living such a life—a kind of end run on medicine—and then dying a quick death. But a recent and very careful study has determined that the idea has no empirical support, and that most of us will contract one or more chronic diseases later in life and die from them slowly. The authors present evidence that between 1998 and 2006, that "at each age over the eight years there is an increase in life expectancy with disease and a decrease in the years without disease. The same is true for functioning loss, an increase in expected years unable to function and a decrease in years able to function." The same, I suspect, might have been said a century ago.

"Health," the study concludes, "may not be improving with each generation.... compression of morbidity may be as illusory as immortality. We do not appear to be moving to a world where we die without experiencing disease, functioning loss, and disability."[9] In a 2006 article the economist David Cutler and colleagues wrote "that the increase in life expectancy beginning at 65 years of age showed the incremental cost of an additional year of life rose from $46,800 in the 1970s to $145,000 in the 1990s. ... If this trend continues in the elderly, the cost-effectiveness of medical care will continue to decrease at older ages."[10] That trend has continued, showing no signs of abatement

Moreover, in thinking about the multiplicity of chronic conditions that can afflict the elderly as they get still older, the longitudinal costs of their care must be taken into account; that is, the costs not of one condition in isolation at a given moment in time, but the cumulative costs over the entire remaining life span of those over 65. It is now possible, and not uncommon, for someone to have cancer at 65, managed heart disease at 75, and Alzheimer disease at 85. If a cure, say, for prostate cancer was discovered and used for someone 65, the probability of some other lethal disease taking its place obviously increases. We don't get out of this world alive. Most of us would probably accept that trade-off in our personal lives, but it is in economic terms a socially expensive one.

In contemplating the recent history of infectious and chronic disease, it ought now to be a reasonable hypothesis that our human physical nature is not nearly as malleable or resilient or open to endless improvement as the research enterprise would like us to believe. In fact, one could say that nature seems to be striking back, first in shattering our belief in the end of infectious disease and paralleling that dismaying defeat with a sturdy resistance to the cure of chronic disease. The great biologist Dubos wrote many years ago in his book *The Mirage of Health* that "complete and lasting freedom from disease is but a dream remembered from imaginings of a Garden of Eden."[11] Had he lived into the present he might have updated that observation by changing "complete and lasting freedom" to "even incomplete and transient freedom from disease." That is what the historical record is beginning to show. While it is not fully clear what the reasons for it are, the decline in drug development raises at least the possibility that some hitherto hidden natural limits may also be appearing.

Average life expectancy, moreover, steadily increasing for many decades, now shows signs of leveling off.[12] S. Jay Olshansky, a leading figure in longevity studies, has for some years expressed skepticism about the prospect of an indefinite increase in life expectancy. He calls his position a "realist" one, particularly in contending that it will be difficult to get the average beyond 85. He also writes that it is "biased" to assume that "only positive influences on health and longevity will persist and accelerate."[13] That view encompasses a belief that medical technologies and science will surely keep movement on a positive track. Not necessarily. For 2010 it was reported that average American life expectancies declined for the first time in many years.[14]

There are many ways of responding to this pessimistic reading of medical progress in recent years. The most common is simply to note all the progress that has been made and is beneficial: useful new drugs, helpful new devices, decreased disability, and so on. An impressive list can be draw up. I am the beneficiary of a life-saving heart operation, of a kind that did not exist a decade ago. But this paper has been examining the macro-trends and developments, the most general of all catalogues of health and illness. That kind of examination yields a far more sobering picture than looking at the micro-level and listing all the good things that have happened.

A no less common response is to say that, however long and difficult the search, there is no reason to believe that the search for cures to infectious and chronic disease may not eventually be found; it is just taking longer than expected and the necessary knowledge for breakthroughs is steadily being accumulated. Hope, in a word, remains a valuable and trustworthy virtue. The fact, moreover, that more people are living longer lives though sick is itself a not inconsiderable triumph. Lives are being saved by those expensive AIDS treatments, just as many of us who would have died earlier from cancer and heart attack can now be saved to live on (my own case).

Those are reasonable responses saved for two considerations. One of them is that, at some point, hope for the future is open to skepticism when too many earlier predictions and prophecies fail to materialize, as has been the case with the eradication of infectious and chronic disease, but not limited to them. Recall also the hoopla over the Human Genome project, whose completion was hailed by Bill Clinton as making it possible to "eradicate once-incurable diseases," and as well the hype that accompanying embryonic stem cell research, opened up in 1998. Opposition to that research, the Alliance for Aging Research said, could harm over 100 million patients in the United States alone.[15] One can observe that already happening in a discreet way by the growing embrace of the idea—call it a kind of tacit truce proposal—that perhaps we should be willing to settle for extending lives with disease rather than hoping to cure them. The other is that the costs of that kind of truce can be prohibitively expensive. It is the wrong kind of truce when it goes on too long and too expensively. We can neither cure them nor afford to pay for chronic disease in its present incarnation: more and more elderly with more and more treatable chronic diseases, but rarely in any low cost way.

In the end, I believe, the cost considerations will begin to trump the trade-off benefits of longer lives in poorer health, now tolerated. While open political discussion of rationing is still off-limits, by politicians anyway, the skirmishes over expensive drug treatments for cancer patients who will gain only a few months of survival time is bound to be expanded even to drugs clearly benefi-cial for much longer survival times; and something similar is likely with high cost heart procedures.

The essence of my argument is that, burdened with the present values and goals of medicine, our health care system is in far deeper trouble than hardly anyone is ready to perceive and take to heart. An abiding faith in medical research and continued open-ended progress is matched by a no less strong belief that a health care system can be devised that can manage whatever that progress brings and whatever its costs. A refrain from some prominent econo-mists is that if medical progress and technological innovation are good "value for money" our society should be ready to pay for it. But value for money is not the same as affordability. It is perfectly imaginable that, if the present tra-jectory of progress against chronic illness is not changed, medicine will be ever more successful in extending the lives of the chronically ill but, if the past track record is any guide, unsuccessful in finding ways to do so economically—which it will have to do in a powerful way to make a decisive difference. Personalized genetic medicine and treatments for breast and prostate cancer that extended life by years and not just months at a cost of $100,000 a patient are not implau-sible medically over the next 30 years. They might well count as good value for money but nonetheless be impossibly expensive for private insurers and public programs to pay for, much less equitably available to everyone who could ben-efit from them.

We have, in short, created a kind of medicine that is economically unafforda-ble in the long run. It is no less a medicine that more or less dooms most of us to lives in our old age that will more often than not end badly, our declining bodies falling apart as they always have, but now devilishly stretching out the pain and decay. Can we conceptualize something better? Can we imagine a medicine 30 years from now that is affordable and thus less ambitious, that handles better the inevitable downward spiral of old age, that helps us through a limited life span, adequately as workers, citizens, and parents? Note that I have already loaded the language of that last question with clues to the direction in which we should go: "less ambitious," "inevitable," "limited," and "adequately."

Here are ten preliminary steps with such an agenda, one which will of necessity require, to use a religious term in a non-religious way, something like a conversion experience on the part of physicians, researchers, industry, and the present.

Step 1: Acceptance of some near certainties: The most important first step is that the hope for decisive cures of infectious and chronic disease must be significantly reduced—it may happen now and then but not much. Infectious disease has not been eliminated, and the cost of care for the chronically ill is certain on its present trajectory to increase the cost of health care well beyond the annual cost-of-living increases. There is no feasible model of health care organization that can effectively control those costs over the long run in other than draconian ways, government- or market-oriented.

Step 2: Devise a fresh concept of medical progress: Vannevar Bush, a distinguished scientific advisor to President Eisenhower, famously said that science is an "endless frontier." He was right then and that is still true now. But scientific progress to extend that frontier is not an endlessly affordable venture. Health care, like the exploration of outer space, will always be open to progress, but we understand that the feasibility of putting humans on Mars is not economically sensible. We have settled for a space station and the Hubble telescope. We must now comparably scale down our ambitions for medical progress, setting new priorities in light of the obstacles encountered with infectious and chronic disease.

Step 3: Setting Research Priorities. The present open-ended model of medical research, with the war against death as the highest priority, should give way to a new goal: aiming to bring everyone up to an average age of 80, already being approached, and shifting the emphasis in the direction of improving the health and quality of life of those under that age. By 80 most people will have lived a full life and death after that age is not ordinarily accounted a human tragedy. The highest priority should be given to the health of children, the next highest those in their adult years, the age group responsible for of managing society, raising children, and caring for the young, and the lowest priority to those over 80.[16]

Step 3: Changing priorities for the elderly. Death is not the worst thing that can happen to the elderly, even if we may yearn for a longer life. An old age marked by disability, economic insecurity, and social isolation are also great evils, probably as threatening as illness and death. Alzheimer disease may never be conquered, and far more necessary for pursuit is development of social support and economic resources to relieve its victims and their families of its burdens. The same can be said of other diseases, such as Parkinson disease, and the frailty of advanced old age, not a disease but an inevitability that is part of aging. Instead of a medical culture of cure for the elderly we need a culture of care and security, notably a stronger Social Security program and a weaker Medicare program.

Step 4: Changing the Rhetoric of Medical Progress. A key ingredient of the economic engine of medical progress has been the endless issuing of promissory notes by scientists and the medical industry, and then broadcast and amplified by the media. The human genome project, stem cell research, and highly touted "breakthroughs" and "promising" new research leads, all continue the rhetorical legacy of the 1970s declaration of a war on cancer. The lives projected to be saved by those advances run, in the aggregate, into the hundreds of millions. They have not materialized. A more realistic rhetoric is necessary, one that places a heavier emphasis on caring for the sick, not curing them.

Step 5: Changing health delivery priorities. Imagine a health care pyramid. At the lowest and broadest level is public health (health promotion and disease prevention); the next level that of primary medicine and emergency care; the level above that of short-term hospital care for acute illness; and the top level that of high-technology care of the chronically ill. The highest priority of health care delivery should be pushing down the ever-expanding kind of care at the highest level to lower levels, and particularly to the public health and primary care levels. The standards for access to care at the highest levels should be severe, marked by a reasonable certainty of a good outcome at a reasonable cost. Cost-effectiveness research and gate-keeping will be necessary to implement that standard. The rise of diabetes, heavily influenced by unhealthy behavior, shows the need for improvement at the public health levels, and a stronger movement toward neighborhood clinics, walk-in access to primary care, and health counseling from an early age on would be imperative. There is no reason to believe that this kind of policy would lower life expectancies, though it might well lower them for elderly patients with late-stage chronic illness and multi-organ failure—which could well be a blessing.

Step 6: Changing the education and acculturation of physicians. Most medical education begins with anatomy, learning from a dead body how it functioned while alive. But the main message of a medical education is to keep people from dying. Yet what if the main message to be learned from the anatomy class is that every patient of every physician will die, and that the task of medicine is only to avert premature death, not death itself. It is instead to make the time between birth and death as healthy as possible, to focus on quality of life not length of life. That latter proposition is by now a cliché, but not one much acted upon. An emphasis of that kind will of course privilege the primary care physician and public health worker, the nurse practitioner and social worker. Higher pay for them and lower pay for specialists will be necessary as well as gate-keeping between primary care and specialist referral. There is nothing new or radical in such a proposal; the disincentives for doing that are enormous. Medical education must be better subsidized to reduce the debt of young physicians, a problem that drives many graduates into specialties. Medicine must be taught, once again, as much of an art as a science, and place the emphasis on population health as much on individual health.

Step 7: Changing industry incentives. The fundamental reality of commercialized American medicine, giving great power to the private sector in determining what to develop and sell, and to determine its price, is that its role in shaping our view of medicine is profound. It caters overwhelmingly to individual needs and desires, and more at the top end of the pyramid than at the lower end. Public health and basic primary care is not where the greatest profit is to be found. The European health care systems have long recognized that the only way to control the commercialization of medicine is by strong government price controls. No other option seems feasible in controlling costs, certainly not competition among suppliers of drugs and devices. If one accepts as a fact, which I do, that the U.S. companies are the main drivers of innovation, thus helping the rest of the world as well, then the main conclusion is that, if innovation is itself one of the leading problems of modern medicine, then all the more reason to impose price controls in this country. Innovation that raises health care costs, in an already overly costly system, is becoming more of a threat than a blessing, and even when it extends life.

Step 8: Changing the public's perception of medicine. The institution of medicine is enormously popular with the public. None of us likes being sick or threatened with death. Modern technological medicine has brought us many benefits that enhance the prestige and social power of medicine. But how can the public be persuaded to lower its expectations of medicine, to more willingly forego expensive chronic care medicine, particularly in old age, and to cast a skeptical eye on the supposed benefits of always pushing back the endless frontier of medical progress? It will, first of all, have to be persuaded to accept something like the seven steps already noted, and the key move in that direction will be for researchers and the media to call repeated attention to the economic and social realities of the endless war on disease: it cannot be won—or can achieve small victories only— and if we are not careful we can harm ourselves trying. The National Institutes of Health study on Alzheimer disease offers a model for such an effort, while the call of President Obama for more research on the disease aiming at a cure is likely to fail (though his call for more social support for caregivers can succeed).

The most important need is to begin a public and professional dialogue on what a new model of medicine will look like—the one we will need 20 years from now. It will be modest in its research aspirations; health care delivery much more heavily financed at the lower end of the pyramid than at the top; dominated by primary care and neighborhood clinics staffed mainly by paramedics for routine health needs and organized teams for acute care; and with many evidentiary barriers to expensive critical care medicine, especially at the end of life. Those who are well will understand that much of their health will depend upon their health-related behavior, that late-life rescue medicine of a kind now available will be much harder to get in the future, that the elderly do not have an unlimited claim on help from the young for expensive medical care, and that the government emphasis will be on stronger social and economic security even at the expense of medical care. Physicians and all allied health professions will have to take the lead in disseminating this information.

9. Changing the health care system. Even if it is successful down to the last detail, the ACA will not succeed in bringing the annual rise in health care costs down to the annual cost-of-living increase. Even on the most optimistic scenario, pushing the insolvency of Medicare back from the earlier projected eight years to 17 years, it will then be back at the brink again, and just when the number of elderly is still rising. How will it make it to the 20 years that I have used for this article?

The long-time problem with Medicare is that it has been held hostage by the background costs of American health care. Unless those costs are controlled, Medicare will still have to face an increase in taxes (when the dependency ratio is worse than today), or cutting benefits (which the ACA will have already done to a considerable degree if its implementation is acceptable). The only reliable way of controlling costs has been the methods used by most other developed countries: a centrally managed government system, control of new and old technologies, price controls, and hospital and national budgets. To be sure, as we now know with those systems, they will also have to shape a fresh view of medicine and its goals (of a kind outlined here or some variant) if they are to control their costs, already under great strain. Only a government managed system can stifle the virus of commercialization, using the provision of medical care as a vehicle for individual and corporate economic gain. Medicine cannot continue trying to serve two masters, that of providing affordable health care and turning a handsome profit for its purveyors and providers.

10. Changing our understanding of health care equality. While it is by no means the case that most Americans believe that everyone should have equal access to affordable health care, a majority does. But there is no way that a fully egalitarian care system can be achieved in 20 years, nor does the model of medicine and health care I propose offer such a promise. Two obstacles, both of which are likely to be permanent, stand in the way. One of them is that, if the care is universal and government-managed, it would have to set limits and ration care to have a budget that was sustainable from one year to the next. That much we can learn from the

European systems, which have severe financial pressures but manage nonetheless to hang on to universal care.

Yet such a move would have two predictable and disturbing consequences: the affluent would be able to buy, at home or abroad, what the government system did not (and could not) provide; and those without such resources would often out of desperation buy care that would financially harm or bankrupt them (which already happens now even with those who have good insurance coverage). It is impossible to imagine any future circumstance that could legally forbid that kind out-of-pocket initiative. In that sense, there will always be a two-tier system. Not even heavily regulated European systems forbid their affluent citizens to go abroad for care they cannot get at home, and all allow the domestic purchase on the private market of medical services not otherwise covered.

There are two solutions to this problem. One of them is to make certain that the government system provides a basic package of care that covers, statistically speaking, a range of services that will satisfy most lifetime needs—"most," that is, not all. The second is that, if the nine other steps proposed above achieve some high degree of success, the excessive demand for health care would decline and the public understanding of high quality care would move toward lower expectations and more realistic hopes. We now have the worst of all combinations, that of an excessively high demand for health care however expensive, and an urgent need to turn back cost escalation. Something has to give there and nothing less than a more austere model of health care will suffice 30 years from now to have an affordable system. That can only be achieved by changing public demands and expectations.

A popular response to this problem is to have private insurers offer a wide range of consumer choices, focusing in particular on the choice of catastrophic care policies for the most expensive illnesses. But there is no reason to believe that unless the present cost escalation of health care was arrested, particularly for chronic illness, that such coverage could remain affordable. And if the out-of-pocket costs before the catastrophic benefits kicked in were themselves at a financially stressful level, the present evidence of the impact of copayments and deductibles shows that, when they are high, people will avoid getting the primary care they need, thus raising the likelihood of higher costs later.

Costs pressure alone as a motive for changing the present progress-intoxicated model of medicine will not by itself be sufficient to motivate public and professional opinion. There are too many self-deceptive ways of evading the likely consequences of uncontrolled cost escalation: faith that research will solve the problem if given time; leaving the hard choices up to individuals in a free medical market; pointing the finger at wasteful practices in other parts of society to show that the money is there if we really need it (as happens in war time with defense expenditures); and the old stand-bys of eliminating waste, inefficiency, fraud and abuse. And that is just a short list of evasive maneuvers. But cost problems provide a catalyst for prodding the public and the professions to ask what kind of medicine will best serve their individual health needs and those of society.

This paper has contended that the open-ended idea of medical progress is itself the main and deepest driver of health care costs, fighting to win an unwinnable war against disease, aging, and death. It no less increasingly dooms us to live too much of our life, especially in our later years, in poor and declining health. Is it really a medical benefit, for ourselves or our families, to live long enough to have a 50% chance of Alzheimer disease, or to be doomed by frailty to a life that makes even walking a hazard? Or to spend our last years in and out of doctor's offices and ICUs as our old age way of life?

Those results are what progress has given us, a seeming benefit that has become a burden, and a way of thinking about medical progress that offers no good way of avoiding that burden. The ten steps listed above give us an alternative. If we do not in some significant degree set about pursuing them, then our medical fate 20 years from now will make the present situation look like a "pleasant spring rain," as a former Director of the Department of Health and Human Services said of the future fate of American health care.[17]

## References

1. Department of Health and Human Services, Administration on Aging, "A Profile of Older Americans: 2010" http://www.aoa.gov/aoaroot/aging_statistics/Profile/2010/4.aspx accessed April 2012.

2. Advert, "HIV and AIDS in America," http://www.avert.org/america.htm; accessed February 2011; Brad Spelberg, *Rising Plague: The Global Threat From Deadly Bacteria and Our Dwindling Arsenal to Fight Them* (Amherst, N.Y.: Prometheus Books, 2009); Martin Enserink, "What's Next for Disease Eradication," (2010) *Science* 330: 1736–1739.

3. Angela B. Mariotto, et al, "Projections of the Cost of Cancer Care in the United States: 2010–2020," (2011) *Journal of the National Cancer Institute* 103 (2): 117.

4. Polo B. Golde, "Cost Trends in Heart Disease, End Stage Renal Disease, Cancer, and Metabolic Syndrome," *Health Care Cost Monitor*, May 22, 2009.

5. National Institutes of Health, State-of-the-Science Conference Statement, "Preventing Alzheimer's Disease and Cognitive Decline," Bethesda, Md.: National Institutes of Health, April 26–28, 2010; Pam Belluck, "With Alzheimer's Patients Growing in Number, Congress Endorses a National Plan," *New York Times*, December 16, 2010.

6. Cited by Kimberly Swartz, "Projected Costs of Chronic Diseases," *Health Care Cost Monitor*, January 22, 2010: Alzheimer's Association, "Alzheimer's Disease Facts and Figures 2007" http://www.alz.org/national/documents/report_2007factsandfigures.pdf.

7. Kenneth E. Thorpe, Lydia L. Ogden, Katya Galactionova, "Chronic Conditions Account for Rise in Medicare Spending from 1987–2006," *Health Affairs* 29 (4): 723.

8. James Fries (1980). "Aging, Natural Death and the compression of Morbidity," *The New England Journal of Medicine* 303: 1369–1370.

9. Eileen M. Crimmins and Hiram Beltran-Sanchez, "Mortality and Morbidity Trends: Is There a Compression of Morbidity?" *Journal of Gerontology: Social Sciences.* 66B (1): 83.

10. David M. Cutler, Allison B. Rosen, and Sandeep Vijan, "The Value of Medical Spending in the United States: 1960–2000," (2006), *The New England Journal of Medicine* 355 (9): 923.

11. Rene Dubos, *Mirage of Health: Utopias, Progress, and Biological Change* (New York; Basic Books, 1979): 2.

12. S. Jay Olshansky, et al, "A Potential Decline in Life Expectancy in the United States in the 21st Century," *The New England Journal of Medicine* (2005) 352: 11.

13. S. Jay Olshansky, "Longevity In The Twentieth Century," *Population Studies* 62 (2): 247

14. Cited by Elizabeth Lopatto, "Life Expectancy in the U.S. Drops for the First Time Since 1993, Report Says" *Bloomberg*, December 9, 2010: Center for Disease Control, "Deaths: Preliminary Data for 2008" *National Vital Statistics Report*, December 2010: vol. 59, no. 2.

15. Cited by Gail Collins, "Public Interests: A Shot in the Dark," *The New York Times,* June 30, 2001: A25;Alliance for Aging Research, "Embryonic Stem Cell Research to Save the Lives of Millions," Spring 2001.

16. Daniel Callahan, *Taming the Beloved Beast: How Medical Technology Costs are Destroying Our Health Care System* (Princeton: Princeton University Press, 2009: see chapter 7, p.171–200.

17. Quoted in Gardner Harris, "British Balance Benefit vs. Cost of New Drug," *The New York Times*, December 3, 2008: A1.

# 15

## TOO MUCH OF A GOOD THING: HOW SPLENDID TECHNOLOGIES CAN GO WRONG

I begin with a brief account of my ordinary workday. Professionally I am engrossed in matters of national health policy, and particularly the growing cost of health care, once again into double digit inflation. Those costs are increasing the number of uninsured, putting great pressure on the federal programs of Medicare and Medicaid, and threatening employer-provided health insurance. What is to be done about that?

To get to my place of work, up the Hudson River, I cross the Tappan Zee Bridge, which is choked with cars, well beyond its original projected capacity, and fed by a highway that features daily traffic jams. What is to be done about that?

The main source of rising health care costs is the emergence of new technologies and the intensified use of old technologies, accounting for some 40% of the annual increase. The main source of the traffic problem, here and elsewhere, is simply too many cars, ever increasing in number. Not many people see analogies between health care technologies and automobiles, but there is nothing like sitting in a traffic jam to expand one's imagination. The problems are more alike than anyone might guess.

Both problems raise two familiar questions, now in a new guise. One is ancient: how should we cope with those features of our lives, and thus of our human nature, where what is good gradually turns into something bad, usually inadvertently? Medical technology is an uncommon human benefit, but when its pursuit and deployment begin to create economic fits, public and private, its good begins to turn bad. The automobile increases freedom and mobility, and like medical technology is a source of enormous national economic benefit. But when our air is besmogged, our highways jammed, and our commutes a misery, its good turns bad.

The second question my two illustrative technologies raise is this: is technology simply a neutral reality, neither good nor bad in itself, but to be evaluated solely on the basis of the uses to which it is put—or does it have a life of its own, subtly shaping our values and ways of life whether we choose that to happen or not? As opponents of gun control are fond of saying "Guns don't kill; only people kill." That may be narrowly true, but is it the full truth? Is it irrelevant for our safety how many guns we have in our house? And are we fully free—the autonomous creatures we are alleged to be—to use or not use medical technology as we like, or to drive or not drive an automobile, or does each technology draw us to its use in ways often beyond our control?

While there are some people who cleverly manage to avoid the health care system altogether, putting their faith in prayer or austere living or exotic jungle potions, most of us can't get away with that. When we hurt we go to the doctor, and doctors these days turn to technology to diagnose us and to treat us. We expect no less. And while there are some strange creatures in Manhattan who have never learned to drive, few of us have successfully evaded the American car culture.

In short, medical technology and the automobile are social realities most of us cannot imagine living without. In each case we can preach moderation; in each, moderation has proved hard to come by. In each case, the cumulative social impact of the technologies seems beyond our control, in great part precisely because it is a good that we cannot easily do without and which (of its very nature?) leads us to want more of it than we now have.

## THE ENDS OF TECHNOLOGY

Technology responds to some deep and enduring human needs: for survival (agriculture, defense); for increased choice, pleasure, and convenience (telephones, movies, escalators); for economic benefit (computers and software, machine tools, airplanes for export); and for liberating visions of human possibility (space travel, instant world-wide communication). Medical technology and the automobile have many if not most of these attractions, and serve most of those needs. And because they serve multiple needs in multiply complex, overlapping ways, their grip on our culture is extraordinarily powerful. Medical technology serves:

- our survival (forestalling death, relieving our morbidities, and softening our disabilities);
- our choice and convenience (with contraception and prenatal diagnosis);
- our economy (jobs, investments, exportable medical equipment and drugs); and
- our dreams of a better, more liberated life (through genetic engineering and psychopharmacology, for example).

No wonder our culture swallows medicine whole. Yet I believe that equity and technological progress are on a profound collision course. The recent rise of health care costs, beginning in the late 1990s, tells the story—depending upon how we look at it. It is tempting to see the problem as strictly technical, solvable by better management, more effective cost control methods, evidence-based medicine, or market solutions that force people to make decisions about what they are willing to pay for. But at base there is a fundamental clash of long-standing values: the golden ideal of unlimited medical and technological progress, at the core of American health care values, versus the social ideal of universal coverage of health care costs, guaranteeing every citizen decent health care at an affordable price. The trajectory of health care costs is rapidly undermining the ideal of affordable, equitable health care, putting universal care in the United States further and further from our grasp.

In thinking about this tension consider a few economic and demographic realities: 40 million uninsured Americans, with the number going up; $1.3 trillion in health care expenditures, the highest in the world and the highest per capita; an increasing array of expensive technologies and drugs; the likelihood that the new genetic-based drugs will be even more expensive than present drugs; inflationary pressures of 10%–20% per year in health care costs over the past couple of years, with no prospect of change in that pattern; an aging population and the imminent retirement of the baby boom generation, likely to push costs even higher; and rising public demands for the latest and the best in medical technology—as the technologies improve, the standards of good health care rise in lock step.

If we are tempted to think that our American problem is unique, it is worth glancing at European and Canadian health care. Those countries long ago embraced universal health care, and for a long time were able to afford it. But they are now hanging on by their nails, subject to the same cost pressures we are. Bit by bit, universal health care in other countries is being eroded: the queues get longer, the out-of-pocket payments increase, denials of care less than urgent become more common. Just as we have, they have tried the efficiency, cut-the-fat route, embraced evidence-based medicine, and even toyed with the idea of health maintenance organizations. Those are all worthy and necessary efforts, but as in the United States, they have not worked well to control costs.

Consider now the automobile. While it does not meet our need for physical survival in quite the way medical technology does, it has proved itself necessary for our:

- social existence (getting where we need to go);
- choice and convenience (going where we want to go, when we want to go there);
- economy (long our leading industry); and
- vision of a better life (living and going where we like).

Yet as with health care, the social and economic costs mount. Some eight million autos were manufactured in 1980, and twelve million in 1999. Americans drove one trillion miles annually in the 1970s, and two trillion by 1999. More is spent on transportation and related costs in the United States than on medical care, education, and clothing combined. The poor can hardly exist without a car to find decent work, and enough has been written about the urban sprawl problem, a product of the car, that I will say nothing more about it.

There is no shortage of solutions to the automobile, but they all have problems. Building more roads is likely to attract more automobiles, eventually using up the initial gains. Improving auto mileage runs into industry opposition. Public transportation is expensive and might not lure people from their autos. Tax incentives and disincentives to control driving patterns might help, but probably won't make a dramatic difference. As with health reform efforts, auto reforms are necessary and sensible—but their chance of putting much of a dent in the overall problem is not encouraging.

What ones sees when comparing medical technology and the automobile is that both serve functions other than those most closely related to their formal ends—health for health care and mobility for the automobile. Those other functions include their economic benefits and their capacity to evoke liberating visions. That combination makes them a far more potent force than if their formal function only was at stake. But those formal functions have proved more than sufficient to give both of them a seemingly unstoppable social force.

It appears, in sum, that both technologies have built within them the capacity to endlessly escalate our desires and raise the baseline of acceptability. Where it was once possible to speak of "the family car," an increasing number of families have individual cars for each person; upscale houses now routinely feature three-car garages. Even if decent public transportation is available, people still want automobiles, and more automobiles.

Here one encounters a puzzle. Is the proliferation of automobiles the result of industry pressures and advertising, or would the desire for cars be there even if those pressures were diminished? I don't know, but my guess is that the natural attraction of the automobile—"natural" in the sense that most adults in most countries will want one—is simply enhanced by advertising and by the symbolic role of the automobile as a token of social status.

One can imagine a limit to the number of cars that the United States might have. If every individual over age sixteen already owned an automobile, then, except for population growth, the number of automobiles would surely level off. And traffic problems could grow so horrendous that people would be fearful of using cars. But one can also imagine the automobile surmounting these limits. Families might acquire more cars than household members, and people might simply become habituated to daily traffic jams—treating them much as they treat the weather, where everyone complains but nobody does anything about it. Everything will then get worse, and we will say it is the price we pay for the benefits.

The situation is far worse with health care. There, the need for good health is in principle unlimited. Our bodies are finite—subject to injury, disease, decline, and death. The best that medicine can do is to ward off those evils, prevent some diseases, rescue us from others, rehabilitate us from still others, and put death off for a time. Medicine can take just pride in the thirty-year increase of average life expectancy in the twentieth century and the rapidly growing number of people living into their 90s and 100s. But eventually something or other gets us.

However great the improvement in health, the doctor's office will still be full and the hospital still a going concern. Put another way, however great medical progress has been, it eventually runs out. We may not encounter the frontier of progress, of medical possibilities, until we are 100, but there is an endless frontier.

With medical technology, it is seemingly impossible to envision some ultimate saturation point. In addition to the endless possibilities of lengthening and improving the human life span, medical research and technological innovation themselves stimulate ideas for even greater future improvements; and with those improvements come greater expectations about what counts as a decent level of health. Scientific progress spurs expectation progress, with the bar always set higher once the earlier goals are achieved. The annual cry during appropriation hearings for the annual National Institutes of Health is that the research promise and possibilities have never been greater; and that is always, in some sense, true. The more we know, the easier it is to know still more.

## GOING TOO FAR

It is easy to understand why we can go too far with the automobile and medical research. In medicine, there is considerable evidence that there is often a "technological imperative" at work, making it hard for physicians, patients, and families to stop treatment with a terminal patient no longer able to benefit from the treatment. So, too, it is possible for individuals to be induced to buy automobiles more expensive than they can afford, or to buy two automobiles when one would do quite nicely.

Medical technology seems to know no boundaries because it is hard to say just what bodily failings and lethal threats we should be willing to accept. The medical research agenda now goes after all lethal diseases, but it also goes after human enhancements and wish fulfillment. Death itself is made to seem an accidental, contingent event. Why do we now die? Not because of the inherent finitude of the human body, as most people thought for most of human history. We die, it is said, because we engage in unhealthy lifestyles, or because research has not yet found a cure for our diseases. And many doctors, when they lose a patient, feel that it is somehow their fault, even if their brain and their colleagues tell them otherwise. For many of our citizens, health has become not simply a necessary means for living a good life, but itself one of the ends of a good life. Medical technology, like the automobile, is imbedded in our culture. It is part of our picture of modern America.

I own a summer house on a small Maine island. When I first went there thirty years ago, there were no more than twenty cars or so. Now there are close to sixty, although the population has not much changed. The island is small and fully walkable; and not long ago everyone did walk, even when they could have driven. The islanders of thirty years ago believed that one of the charms and assets of the island was the absence of cars; and there seems to have been a built-in, culturally transmissible, taboo—a self-imposed limit that kept the cars out. But once the trend toward cars got started, the earlier limits transgressed, little was to stand in their way.

## TECHNOLOGY AS A NEUTRAL FORCE

Given the power of medical technology and the automobile to have such a hold on our lives, I find it hard to say that they are merely neutral tools, to be used or not used as we see fit, just lying about. Except for their pejorative connotations, I find technologies to be much like viruses or germs. They are external agents that can invade our bodies and make a great difference in our fate and health.

But that is to speak in a general way. We also know that even in the worst plagues, not everyone perishes. The social context and the character of individual bodies affect the outcome. This is why we often think of viruses as neutral: they do not behave in any wholly independent, context-free way. Of course, common sense dictates that we treat them with care, avoiding them when possible, but no one is guaranteed to get sick from contact with them.

Medical technology and the automobile are similar. Not everyone will, so to speak, invariably be infected by them, though both are hard to avoid. And just as some diseases that are medical threats to individuals also confer some genetic protection, so too medical technology and the automobile have many valuable traits. Our health depends on the e-coli bacteria in our gut; but outside of that setting, let loose in the world, e-coli can be deadly. I once suggested at a meeting at the Centers for Disease Control and Prevention (CDC) that, in light of the national obesity problem, perhaps a Surgeon General s warning should be affixed to every automobile and TV set, warning of their health dangers if used to excess. Everyone laughed except the director of the CDC. He said that he did not think that was a politically promising way to go, and I came away with the impression that even as a joke it was impermissible. Similarly, when I even suggest to most audiences, much less to research advocates, that we might want to rethink and even slow down and redirect innovation in medical technology, I am guaranteed a chilly, shocked reaction.

In sum, if in some literal sense technology is neutral, in the important sense of the way it affects human lives it is anything but neutral. When the technology is ubiquitous, when it serves important human values and ways of life, and when it is all but impossible to avoid using, then it has captured our lives. Most new technologies are introduced not as enslaving tyrants, but as choice-increasing, society-enhancing developments that we are free to take or leave. But as the rise and dominance of the automobile and medical technology show, freedom and choice can be fleeting when the technology takes up a central place in our cultural gut and we require them as much as our private gut requires e-coli.

I will conclude by noting that with both technologies there are alternatives. A few years ago in Prague I was talking with a doctor who often had to spend her weekends at the hospital where she worked. She always took the tram rather than driving the family car. When I pointed out that it was a ten-minute ride by car, with plentiful parking available, but forty-five minutes by tram, she looked at me in an uncomprehending way and said, in effect, that she could not understand why anyone would drive anywhere when public transportation was available.

In the case of medical technology, it is well known that most of the improvements in health status have come from public health measures and improved socioeconomic status. Much more research is needed on the background conditions and determinants of health, but the big research money goes to genetic and other biomedical research, looking into the depths of biology for cures rather than into the breadth of human societies to determine why some people get sick and others do not. This latter approach—often called a population rather than individual perspective—has powerful theoretical support. What it does not have is glamour, an economic lobby, and an intuitive appeal equivalent to the development of new technologies.

The difficulty with these alternative strategies with the automobile and medical technologies is that they have not sunk into our public and private psyche with the power of the technologies. They do not have behind them the overlapping strands of attraction and profit that the technologies do. They do not—to recur to my language above—seem to have the power to change our way of life, to bury themselves so deeply within our way of life that, however much we worry and complain about their harms, we cannot let go of the good and goods they bring.

Could all of that change? Maybe. It may be that the health care cost problem will become so bad that the now well-insured middle class will begin to hurt, and will consider some serious alternatives. It may be that the traffic jams and commutes will grow so long that the public will revolt against the hegemony of the automobile. In other words, for those of us looking for a change, probably the best we can hope for is a nasty crisis that will *force* a change. But it's not likely to happen. As those of us who have longed for universal health care for many decades long ago learned, the capacity of this country to muddle through what in other places would seem a great crisis is formidable.

*Acknowledgments*

This article is based on a lecture given in May 2002 at MIT as The Morison Lecture and Prize in Science, Technology and Society.

# 16

---

# DEMYTHOLOGIZING THE STEM CELL
# JUGGERNAUT

The national debate on embryonic stem cells and research cloning has brought out the best and the worst in American culture. The best is on display in many ways. It is a debate that has been marked by an outpouring of sympathy for those suffering from disease or disability or threatened with death. It has drawn on the deep historical reservoir in America of a devotion to research and technological innovation to relieve the human condition. Despite these intensely partisan times, support for the research has easily crossed party lines, among legislators and the public. And it has given hope to perhaps thousands of people suffering from tenacious afflictions and disabilities. Those elements of the debate are impressive and commendable.

Far less commendable were many of the ways in which the campaign in favor of the research was waged to gain money to carry it out. The main focus of this paper is on the early years of the stem cell debate when that effort was most intense. There were, for openers, inflated claims about the value of the research, often in the face of cautions from the researchers themselves. There was also an egregious promotion of what I believe to be an utterly wrong view about a so-called moral obligation to pursue the research. And there was a full display of that most ancient of logical fallacies, the *ad hominem* argument. Many research proponents did not hesitate to label those on the other side as a noxious coalition of right-wing religious fanatics, the fearful, the superstitious, the ignorant, and those invincibly indifferent to human suffering. Some of that kind of rhetoric has been thrown in my direction. The right, sometimes not to be outdone in throwing mud, labeled proponents as enemies of human dignity, who were well down a slippery slope to manufacturing and instrumentalizing human embryos and thus life itself, the crudest kind of utilitarianism.

There may have been bits of truth in each of these stereotypes, but they did not serve well to advance the discussion. There were some larger issues at stake in this conflict, most notably the excessive hype and hyperbole deployed by research supporters, the use of bad arguments, some ethical window-dressing to move the cause along, and a failure to take account of some little-noted but highly relevant facts.

I confess at the outset that I oppose embryonic stem cell research for either research or human cloning purposes. It is by now evident that I was on the losing team and, as someone who thinks of himself as a liberal, I found myself in the company of many whose values I do not share. I also happen to be pro-choice on abortion, which probably puts me in some odd, idiosyncratic class, maybe a class of one.[1] I will try to reconcile this combination later in the paper.

I most want to demythologize the stem cell juggernaut. The late Protestant theologian Rudolf Bultmann used the term "demythologize" as a way of describing his effort to downplay or altogether deny some key beliefs of Christianity, but without altogether rejecting Christianity. Analogously, I want to deflate the case made for research cloning but not for, say, adult stem cell research (even if it is less "promising"). I use the term "juggernaut" to convey my perception that the force of the research drive, and the public relations work that was invested in it, were remarkable. If it did not persuade President George W. Bush to change his mind, it has otherwise swept away most other opposition. President Barack Obama has already lifted some of the restrictions on the limited use of embryos now in place in government-supported research, although further Congressional action is needed before federal funding may be used in the creation of new cell lines.[2] The fact that many states, some of them facing large budget problems, decided to support the research is just one piece of testimony about the intensity of the enthusiasm. These states include California, Connecticut, Illinois, and Wisconsin.[3]

## I. IS THERE A MORAL OBLIGATION TO DO EMBRYONIC STEM CELL RESEARCH?

I begin with the leading candidate for demythologization—the claim that there is some kind of powerful and inescapable moral obligation to carry out the research.

## A. Considerations that Weigh Against a Moral Obligation

Well before the stem cell era, the Nobel Laureate Joshua Lederberg once said to me that "the blood of those who will die if biomedical research is not pursued will be upon hands of those who do not support it." Much more recently the distinguished stem cell researcher, Irving Weissman, used almost identical language on behalf of stem cell research. According to this line of thought, regenerative medicine has the promise and potential of saving millions of lives, afflicted by conditions from heart disease to Alzheimer disease, from diabetes to Parkinson disease. There is said to be a "negative responsibility" for the lives of those that could be lost in the absence of the research.

What a rhetorical club to use—but this claim seems specious and bombastic.[4] I advance three considerations to support my view. The first is that there is a common impression that stem cell research holds out the only hope of curing various prominent diseases—heart disease, diabetes, Alzheimer and Parkinson disease, and spinal cord injury. Not so. The National Institutes of Health has invested tens of billions of dollars to cure or ameliorate exactly those same diseases over the years; and it now invests at least $2.8 billion on them each year.[5] The private for-profit sector has invested at least that much as well, and of course each of those diseases has an advocacy group that raises additional research money. Unless we think that the private and public research sectors are simply squandering their money, which no one has said, and unless we believe that none of that ongoing research is "promising" (the most oft-repeated term with stem cell research), then it is simply wrong to assert that the omission of research cloning would amount to an egregious indifference to human suffering.

Many scientists and others say that embryonic stem cell research is the most promising approach. But no one (so far as I know) has even dared to offer statistical probabilities of eventual success, and many are willing to concede that there may never be a dramatically effective clinical application (though they usually add that there will be great gains in basic knowledge).[6] In sum, if there is a moral obligation to do medical research on various deadly diseases, that obligation is already being discharged. To say that the omission of *one* line of research among many others, embryonic stem cell research, constitutes a moral failure of the first magnitude—"blood on our hands"—is insupportable. But it certainly plays well.

The second consideration bears on what economists call "opportunity costs": that is, what else might usefully be done with the money going into stem cell research? At the same time that the $3 billion California referendum was being debated, for instance, the newspapers in that state were reporting that 2.2 million (mainly immigrant) adults were functionally illiterate, almost certainly dooming them to poverty, low level jobs, and little upward mobility.[7] The spending of

$3 billion on educating them would produce certain and not just promising social benefits, definite and not just speculative community gains—unlike the speculative clinical gains from stem cell research. But no celebrities, leading scientists, biotechnology entrepreneurs, prominent businessmen, or politicians proposed any referendum on that problem. Nor have many of the states initiating stem cell research, sometimes into the hundreds of millions of dollars, been hesitant about simultaneously cutting back on Medicaid benefits, as if the future benefits for future sick people are more important than present benefits for present people.

The third consideration bears on medical progress and medical need. Proponents of the research treat illness and disease as the greatest of threats to human welfare. I would say they are serious harms but by no means the worst facing our society. Even more threatening are the failures to provide insurance for those who do not have it, various forms of inequitable distribution of available resources of many kinds, global warming, racial and immigrant prejudices, poor support of working mothers, and many of the harms that were done to our society by the Bush administration's threats to civil liberties and sensible social priorities.

The developed countries of the world, including the United States, have an average life expectancy (accounting for male and female differences) of about seventy-seven years. This level of life expectancy is perfectly sufficient to sustain generally healthy, economically successful societies. The fact that heart disease (a stem cell target) is our nation's leading killer in no sense entails that it should be considered a major societal problem—unless anything and everything people die from should be considered a national disaster.

In spite of these indicators of disordered priorities, recent conventional research and improved clinical care are, for instance, steadily reducing heart disease mortality. The greatest threat of diabetes does not now come about only from the lack of a cure, but by increasing obesity, a far harder problem to deal with than inadequate treatments. It is also obvious that most of the stem cell target diseases are, save for diabetes and spinal cord injuries, diseases of aging societies, with heart disease, cancer, and increasingly Alzheimer disease at the top of the list. Unless we think it an inherent evil that people die in old age, and that nothing less than all-out warfare is required to stamp out diseases that primarily afflict them, then it is reasonable to give a lower research priority to them.

As far as I can make out, the most evil events of the twentieth century came from man's inhumanity to man—world wars, genocide, racial and ethnic violence—not from death by disease, save in poor countries, which are often bereft of research on those tropical and other diseases (such as malaria) that kill them. I believe there is an obligation to carry out research on those tropical diseases as well as HIV/AIDS, which destroys young lives and civic infrastructures in a way far worse than any disease that might be cured or ameliorated by regenerative medicine.

None of the considerations I have offered tell against stem cell research as such, simply against the use of embryos as research material. Adult stem cell research is fine, and if a way can be found to gain embryonic stem cells without destroying embryos that is fine as well. Although I do not believe there is any moral duty to advance the research, to do so could still be considered a human *good*, well worth a public and private investment. But if it is characterized as a good, not an overriding obligation, then it must pass the test of competition and comparison with other goods that need to be pursued for the sake of a better society. What I reject is the high pedestal on which it has been set. For a yet-unproven research possibility, stem cell research does not deserve that honor—though it surely helps to raise money and generate publicity.

### B. The Campaign in Support of Stem Cell Research: Origins of a "Moral Duty"

How did embryonic stem cell research get put on such a high pedestal? Historians may someday aptly characterize the drive on behalf of stem cell research as "the perfect PR campaign," one of the best ever waged for medical research. This campaign began in 1998 with a rash of media stories about James Thomson's derivation of the first embryonic stem cell lines from frozen human embryos.[8] Those stem cells, the public was told in often breathless ways, hold the promise of a whole new medical field, that of regenerative medicine, restoring damaged or destroyed cells in many organs of the body.

But it soon became evident that there would be opposition to the research— and particularly against federal support of it—mainly from conservative quarters. At that point the advocates ratcheted up the campaign. Its organizers, led by well-funded research advocacy organizations and various scientific societies, turned to the tried and true methods pioneered in the 1950s by two wealthy philanthropists, Mary Lasker and Florence Mahoney, at that time on behalf of larger appropriations for the National Institutes of Health. Their key tactics were to put together a coalition of prominent scientists, politicians, business people, and celebrities; amass a war chest to pay for publicity; and skillfully use the media.[9] It was a tactic that worked well in the 1950s, and it worked no less well as the 1990s drew to a close and the new millennium arrived. It also had an added touch, which did not hurt. Bush's rejection turned out to be, among Bush critics, an added benefit: if he did not like it, there must have been something going for it.

The Alliance for Aging Research set the tone with its much-cited claim that up to 150 million lives could (and would, and should) be saved if the research was allowed to go forward.[10] Thomas Okarma, CEO of the leading biotechnology firm, Geron, said that "not to develop the technology would do great harm to over 100 million patients in the U.S. alone." A powerful endorsement of the research by dozens of Nobel laureates from all fields of science was publicized,[12] as was a comparable statement of 100 college presidents[13] (most of whom, it is fair to assume, are hardly expert on the subject). Highly supportive public opinion surveys were released, as were enthusiastic declarations by prominent federal senators and representatives. Christopher Reeve, Michael J. Fox, and the journalists Michael Krondack and Michael Kinsley, each the victim of one of the target diseases, played the celebrity role. The National Academy of Sciences and the Institute of Medicine provided glowing endorsements. The media had no trouble finding stories about desperate parents hoping for a cure to their child's diabetes, or spouses taking care of Alzheimer disease patients, or paraplegics trapped in wheelchairs. The real estate tycoon behind the push for the California bond initiative, Robert N. Klein, spoke perfectly the inflated language of the national campaign, calling the discovery of the potential of stem cells "one of the great watershed discoveries in history."[14]

It soon became hard to find many in my field, bioethics, who spoke out against the research. As a well-known journalist once asked me, "Why are bioethicists in such lock-step on this issue?" I could think of no answer that would not bring further embarrassment to a field that likes to think of itself as open, evenhanded, and non-partisan. Cynicism greeted the appointment of Leon R. Kass, a longstanding opponent of both reproductive and research cloning, to chair President Bush's Council on Bioethics. That appointment was railed against in the press and in bioethics chat rooms, treated as nothing more than a far-right move to put an ethical polish on an intolerable, ideology-driven hostility to life-saving research. The columnist Robert Kuttner spoke out against the religious dogmatists standing in the way of the research.[15] No such label is attached to those religious figures who oppose the war in Iraq.

Notably missing from the campaign was any recollection of some earlier advocacy efforts, each accompanied by excitement, hostility toward conservative critics, and unbounded hopes. Well over a decade ago there was a similarly controversial effort to support the implantation of fetal tissue in the brains of Parkinson patients. It failed, and decisively so. Then there was the effort, beginning around the same time, to test gene therapy as a means of curing disease. That therapy has had meager results and, along the way, claimed the life of a research subject, Jesse Gelsinger.[16] But no letdown seemed quite as striking as that following the completion of the highly touted $3 billion effort to map the human genome, the Human Genome Project. Bill Clinton celebrated the end of that effort by saying it would now be possible to "eradicate once-incurable diseases."[17] Such talk is muted these days. It turns out that there are many fewer human genes than projected, and that in any case proteins—the delivery system for genetic expression—may be more important for medical applications than genes alone. The mantle of eradicating "once-incurable diseases" has now been passed to stem cell research.

There is a scientific response to stories of that kind. Each of the cited failures or disappointments may not, in the long run, turn out to be failures after all. Good science takes time, with many disappointments along the way. The contention that adult stem cells, which can be harvested without embryo destruction, may be as promising as embryonic stem cells regularly draws a brisk response: the embryonic form looks theoretically more promising but, whatever view turns out to be right, good science wants to go down *all* available roads, never knowing in advance which will eventually work best. No doubt that kind of general argument about scientific progress is, historically taken, perfectly true. It is also no less true that it has provided cover for outlandish and improbable scientific promises and possibilities.

I raise the issue of hype, however, not as an argument against the research. Its real harm is that it feeds the notion of a "negative responsibility" or a "moral obligation" to pursue the research. That latter is an argument meant to disarm critics, to overcome ethical objections and resistance, and to characterize opponents as immoral or soft on human suffering. George W. Bush, ironically, must have been reading the same rhetorical playbook by calling the terrorism problem a threat to our "national security," and the fight against it a "war." And those who oppose the "war" are, to be sure, labeled as unpatriotic at best and indifferent to the suffering imposed by terrorists at worst.

What about the present case: excessive hype or reasonable hope? The common sense answer is that it is too early to know. But there have been many warning flags along the way, almost always buried at the end of media stories that headline new mouse breakthroughs, further lives to be saved, hopes for support from the new administration, and voices of indignation at the foot-dragging of George W. Bush (for whom, it should be noted, I did not vote). Yet even the most hopeful of scientists have been saying since 1998 that turning the research promise into useful clinical applications, if possible at all, could take years or even decades to accomplish.

The May 2005 announcement that South Korean researchers had created new lines of embryonic stem cells that, for the first time, carry the genetic signature of diseased or injured patients, and which can be derived in fewer than twenty tries, signaled a great increase in efficiency.[18] It was hailed by other scientists as a dramatic and spectacular advance. Yet it all turned out to be a fraud and an acute embarrassment to the research community. But, if anything, too much was made of it. Fraud has always been present in science. The main importance of the South Korean case was to demonstrate that a well-hyped campaign, with glittering prizes at the end, invites abuse: the greater the prize, the greater the temptation.

Yet at more or less the same time, in June of that year, James Thomson, while continuing to call for federal support of the research, laid out a number of cautions in an interview, in addition to the common scientific reservations about the long time it will take to get any useful clinical results. He said, as the interviewer summarized his comments, "that supporters of stem cell research are overestimating the prospects for transplantation cures, that the current stem-cell lines [and not just those authorized by President Bush, but new ones as well] are not well-suited for such applications anyway, and that there's no need to resort to therapeutic [research] cloning now—or perhaps ever."[19]

While I am not competent to assess his scientific views, it is noteworthy that he had a good word to say for President Bush's compromise position: "[I]t did get the field started, and I think that's a positive way of looking at it."[20] However, he also echoed a frequent criticism of opposition to stem cell research: "[M]ost of the people who oppose this research, and most of those who support this research, do it with a profound amount of misinformation.... [Everyone should have] real facts."[21] Well, what should we know? Thompson's interview was interlaced with what he acknowledged to be guesses, uncertain predictions, and varying future scenarios. What facts, if any, would make the prognostication more reliable? For the future of financial and political support, it is important to assess the future of the research. We need to know whether it is a good bet or not, and so far that remains uncertain. There have been, as of 2008, no striking breakthroughs on the clinical front, and the fact that some prominent researchers are now saying that the greatest gain may come from the knowledge generated rather than for the cure of disease may be telling a different story than the one initially advanced. The first clinical trial using cells derived from embryonic stem cells was announced in 2009 (though there was controversy about whether this trial was premature).[22]

It is a fact that a great deal of money and energy, and the best of American public relation and advocacy skills, has been invested in the selling of stem cell research, particularly the embryonic kind. As the California bond drive demonstrated, a combination of biotechnology entrepreneurs, wealthy real estate tycoons, grant-seeking scientists, a muscular governor and other leading politicians, and an eager public have deeper pockets for advocacy than even the Southern California religious right. In the United States, any cause that proclaims improved health and the conquest of disease is usually an easy winner in ideological combat, especially if its cause is pressed with big money and media savvy, and given medical credibility by credentialed experts.

## II. EMBRYOS, EMBRYOS, AND MORE EMBRYOS: THEORIES ON THE PERSISTENT DISAGREEMENT OVER THE MORAL STATUS OF THE EMBRYO

I now turn to the moral status of the embryo. For about thirty-five years now I have puzzled and struggled over that status. Some people have sublime and calm self-confidence in the rightness of their views on this issue, and this trait seems to be evenly displayed on the right and left. There is also persistent perplexity on the part of many others—that is, most of us. Wherever one stands, however, it might readily be agreed that there is no end of the disagreement in sight. I have puzzled about why it is hard to achieve consensus. As my wife (prolife) and I (prochoice) long ago noted, after decades of argument, we each know all the relevant science and all the relevant moral and philosophical arguments; it is hard to find anyone who can say anything new to either of us. Still, we disagree. I have three theories about this difficulty of overcoming disagreement: one bears on our interests and self-interests, another on our modes of moral analysis, and the third on devising public policy and a regulatory framework for research.

### A. Interests and Self-interests

My way of understanding the methodological problems of determining the moral status of the embryo, which has helped me to see why there is no decisive general method of solving problems that mix scientific evidence and moral evaluation, has ineluctably (and sometimes unpleasantly) led me to consider the role played in the process by our interests and self-interests. There are two ways of framing the problem I want to point to. One of them has been to ask why it is that the passions run so high for pro-life and pro-choice advocates in the abortion wars. Each of them has, in my observation, invested their stand with symbolic and policy considerations that go beyond abortion and the moral standing of embryos (or fetuses). Let me call this the "interest" problem: important matters are at stake, bearing on what each side sees as the kind of world in which they want to live, and the only kind of world that anyone should want to live in.

For many feminists, abortion has been a decisive index issue, one whose outcome determines what women's role and social status will be in many areas other than reproduction. If we lose that battle, they have in effect said, we will have lost the war for women's rights. For pro-life advocates, the moral status of embryos and fetuses is no less a decisive index issue, determining how we think of and treat the weakest and most defenseless among us. If we lose this battle, they are saying, we will have lost the war for human dignity. At the extremes, some pro-choice feminists say that the moral status of embryos and fetuses is solely a matter of a woman's decision: they have value insofar as women confer value on them—and that is the kind of absolute power women should have. For their part, some pro-life proponents want abortion, however early the stage, to be understood as nothing less than murder of the innocent, justifying for some violence and non-peaceful protest against those who carry out such atrocities. These attitudes are mainly found at extreme edges of the abortion struggle, but they are less surprising (if not less disturbing) when it is understood that there are larger causes and concerns at stake, of which the moral status of the fetus is the tinderbox, not the whole story.

What I will call the "self-interest" problem raises a number of delicate puzzles. By this I mean the extent to which people, wittingly or unwittingly, allow their self-interest to determine their moral judgments. If my reading of the methodological problem of determining the moral status of the embryo is plausible—we lack any decisive criteria for making a decision—the self-interest issue must consequently raise its head. The way is open, and it is a wide avenue, for the introduction of ideological, political, and self-interested judgments. That is what patently appears to happen.

At least two senses of self-interest can be distinguished. One of them is what might be called acceptable or legitimate self-interest: a minority group seeking an end to discrimination against itself, the disabled lobbying for access to public facilities, or homeowners seeking the end of industrial pollution practices that threaten their water supply or the health of their children. Each group seeks something of direct benefit to them, perhaps of no particular benefit to the rest of the community, and perhaps even imposing some burdens on everyone else—but it is considered a legitimate claim and a tolerable burden even on those who have nothing special to gain.

But then there is what I will call an ambiguous sense of self-interest, which might be those situations where we at least wonder if the self-interest is crass, that is, where narrowly self-serving desires are at stake. Here we might think of the industrial polluter who knows that there is hazardous pollution that it could well afford to stop. But it persuades itself that the pollution is not all that bad, that nature will eventually take care of it as it biodegrades, and that any serious efforts on its part would endanger its economic strength and thus put at risk the many jobs the community needs. I stress in this example that the company "persuades itself," in order to recognize that most people who display crass self-interest may admit that some self-interest is at stake but not the grossly self-serving kind.

What are we to make of embryonic research scientists who, we assume, must have persuaded themselves that embryos do not have a high enough moral status for concern, and maybe none at all, and thus see no problem in using them for their research? Is it a mere coincidence that, seemingly, only a handful of scientists interested in doing the research appear to have any serious dilemma about using embryos, a far lower proportion than the population as a whole? This can be seen as a classic chicken-egg problem: which came first, their desire to do the research and thus an adaptation of their moral stance toward embryos through self-persuasion; or was there a preexisting stance toward embryos that made it morally tolerable to use them for research?

The same kind of questions can be raised about the lay supporters of the research and particularly those suffering from some disability or life-threatening disease that the research might alleviate. At the least we might say that, for those who want the research to go forward, there are some powerful disincentives against granting embryos so high a status that the research could not proceed. Or, to put it a different way, if the destruction of embryos is understood to be one of balancing their value against that of research benefits, it is not exactly unpredictable that many people will persuade themselves that embryos have a lesser value than those benefits.

I focus on this line of thought because, if science cannot tell us what the moral status of an embryo is, and therefore if the moral values at stake must, so to speak, be imported from the outside, then there is room to seek those moral principles and modes of reasoning most compatible with our other values. If we are as scientists eager to carry out the research, and as patients eager to have its benefits, we will be likely to bring those values to bear on our assessment of embryos—and to decide against them. But my mode of analysis here cuts two ways: for those who see in various forms of scientific research a threat to human dignity (an important value for their way of life) or the beginning of a slippery slope, they have a powerful incentive to give the embryo a high and inviolable status.

I do not conclude from my line of analysis that the obvious self-interest of either the researchers or their opponents is a matter of crass self-interest; however, I also do not believe that either group is disinterested. The scientific interests of researchers (their notions of the goods to be pursued) are best served by minimizing the moral status of embryos, just as the moral interests of opponents (their notions of the higher goods at stake) are served by maximizing it. What all of this proves to me is that the ambiguous status of the embryo—inescapable since it requires a mode of combined scientific/moral analysis for which we have no good methods—invites and perhaps makes necessary the introduction of values and perspectives drawn from other ways of understanding what we take to be the human good; and these values and perspectives open the way for a self-interested stance. It only gets crass when our own view of what that good might be is utterly self-serving. I do not hesitate to ascribe this judgment to the view of some feminists that the value of the embryo depends entirely on the value a woman chooses to confer upon it, or to politicians who boorishly court conservative support for their election by pandering to pro-embryo forces, treating their enemies as killers.

## B. Moral Analysis, Uneasiness, and "Respect": Deriving an "Ought" from an "Is"

There persists a widespread conviction that the answer to the status of the embryo can be found in science. Hence, there are endless debates about the embryological evidence, about whether one can speak of a pre-embryo, about whether human life could someday be derived from a single skin cell, about whether more scientific evidence might one day solve the problem, and so on. But to ask about the moral status or standing of an embryo is an ethical question, and if there was ever an instance when it is not possible logically to derive an *ought* from an *is* (known to philosophers as the naturalistic fallacy), this is it.

Science may eventually be able to empirically explain everything to be known about embryos, their genesis, and their development. But it is beyond the capacity of science to tell us how we ought to treat embryos or evaluate their moral status. That evaluation falls into the category of issues that requires a blend of empirical analysis and moral judgment, but each mode of reasoning draws upon different methods and standards of judgment. To further complicate matters, those different forms of judgment can influence each other: our moral concerns can lead us to look at one among many aspects of the scientific evidence, selecting those that seem relevant (itself a non-scientific judgment), while the scientific evidence can lead us to reconsider our moral judgments, sometimes whether we like it or not.

Could one conclude from my analysis above that there is nothing more to an evaluation of the moral status of the embryo than our various interests and self-interests at play and manifesting our different views of the good life? There are surely some grounds for thinking so, but there are some reasons to hesitate as well. While there are many research proponents who seem to believe that embryos have no value whatever, they seem to be in the minority. I characterize the stance of many if not most proponents as one of uneasiness, displaying some residual uncertainty about the status of embryos. This uneasiness seems to me to come out in a number of ways: an acknowledgement that, if implanted and not destroyed, embryos have the potential to develop into full persons; a reluctance, other than as a last resort, to create embryos solely for research purposes; an aversion to commercializing the use of embryos, and finally by the adoption of the word "respect" as an apparent effort to find a symbolic compromise characterization of what we owe embryos.

Just what is it that bothers people, even those readily willing to trade off embryos for valuable research? I cannot say for sure, but I suspect that, however much some philosophers may deride the importance of potentiality ("acorns are not oak trees, are they?"), it is hard to entirely put out of our mind and emotions that we all began as embryos; undeniably they are part of everyone's personal history. Even if, as is customary, a distinction is made between the beginning of individual life, on the one hand, and protectable moral standing on the other, that beginning is hard to ignore.

But I can only speculate about the sources of the uneasiness. I want to take a look instead at the word "respect," a much-employed way of placating and domesticating the discomfort. A 1979 report of the Ethics Advisory Board of the Department of Health, Education, and Welfare stated that the early embryo merits "profound respect," though not all "the full legal and moral rights attributed to persons."[23] A 1994 NIH Human Embryo Research Panel said that "the preimplantation human embryo warrants serious moral consideration as a developing form of human life."[24] The National Bioethics Advisory Commission said in 1999 that "human embryos deserve respect as a form of human life."[25]

Since the context of that usage of "respect" is that of the destruction of the embryo, this amounts to what I would call cosmetic ethics. The dictionary definitions of "respect" appear to leave little room for its use as a balm to the conscience, demanding something more of us than a deferential nod in their direction as they are destroyed strictly for our ends, not their own. Their death is certain, the research results wholly speculative. Try fitting the notion of respect as used by the various commissions into the standard dictionary definitions of respect: "1. To feel or show esteem for; to honor; 2. To show consideration for; avoid violation of; treat with deference."[26]

How can I criticize this symbolic deference paid to embryos and, at the same time, defend the legalization of abortion? In the most defensible abortions, for a serious threat to a woman's health or the certain likelihood of a crippling genetic defect for her embryo or fetus, an abortion can have almost certain beneficial results, at least from the perspective of a woman who believes that it is necessary. Hence, the destruction of the embryo (or, much more likely, a fetus) in that case brings an almost certain benefit to a woman: a life is taken but another life gains, and in that case a life already fully developed gains, not hypothetical future patients who may, in any event, be cured by means of research other than the use of stem cells. I would not want to call the destruction of the embryo or fetus in that case a respectful act, even for a defective fetus. This is still destruction pure and simple, but for very different reasons than clinical research. In short, a different kind of case can be made for abortion, with equally deadly results, than can be made for embryo research. An acceptance of abortion does not entail an acceptance of embryo destruction for research purposes.

## C. Public Policy: Embryonic Stem Cell Alternatives, Excess Embryos, and Regulation of Research

I have already tried to make the case that there is no moral obligation to pursue embryonic stem cell research, particularly in light of the vast amount of money already being spent to combat the same conditions at which the research is aimed. Whether the various ideas for deriving stem cells by means other than embryo destruction will succeed is uncertain at this writing, but it would appear to be a worthy goal. That very effort has been challenged on the grounds that there are already thousands of frozen embryos available for research, otherwise to be discarded. That is a tantalizing argument, hard to resist because of its common-sensical nature. Even so, on balance I do resist it, but for a cluster of reasons, not one in particular.

Excess frozen embryos exist as a result of in vitro fertilization, which in itself seems to me perfectly acceptable. Must less acceptable are the reasons why there are so many frozen embryos available. Most of them come from the treatment of infertile women, but most (though not all) of those women are infertile because of two well-known causes, late procreation and sexually transmitted infection. I would classify excess embryos, then, as a public health problem—yet one that we have medicalized as an inherent biological problem, to be clinically treated rather than the subject of efforts to change the underlying cause (particularly creating social and economic contexts that encourage women to procreate earlier rather than later, in their twenties rather than thirties).[27] Of late, it might be mentioned, efforts are underway to improve in vitro fertilization to reduce the number of spare embryos, and of course there have been many scientific doubts about whether many or most frozen embryos would be useful anyway.[28] I will not take up here the effort to find ways of gaining stem cells without destroying embryos, but it is an obviously useful effort.

26. The American Heritage Dictionary of the English Language 1107 (1st ed. 1969). I am not greatly impressed with the argument that spare embryos will be destroyed anyway, and that their use in research is better than simply wasting them. I come to that judgment for a variety of reasons, not one of which is (even to me) fully persuasive in itself, but which add up to a moral gestalt that tilts me against that use: 1) spare embryos need not, and should not exist in the first place—they enhance the chances of an eventual pregnancy, but do not guarantee it, and the recent efforts to reduce their number reflects, at least in part, some level

of discomfort; 2) research on dying human beings without their informed consent was once accepted in medical research on the grounds that they were dying anyway and it would be a waste not to make use of them; 3) the one-time (now defrocked) champion of euthanasia, Dr. Kevorkian, contended that the organs of those who were going to suffer capital punishment should routinely be salvaged without their consent because, after all, they were going to be dead soon, and thus would have no further use for their organs and that—clincher of clincher—the salvaged organs could save lives (and Chinese penal authorities have used an identical argument); and 4) the Nazi doctors, who did all kinds of horrible things to concentration camp inmates prior to their certain death in the name of medical research, consoled themselves with the thought of all the medical benefits that could accrue from enlisting the inmates without consent. The research was mainly useful for militarily valuable purposes but at least some seems to have been for saving lives in general. Do we want contemporary medical research placed in such unsavory company? As I said, there is a response to each of the points (we're not Nazis, Chinese penal authorities, or Kevorkian—just good people trying to reduce suffering and death), but their net weight leaves a bad odor in the room, too much for me, at any rate. I would be more impressed with Gene Outka's argument based on a "nothing is lost" principle if I believed it legitimate to have spare embryos, which I do not (it is not medically necessary), and if I believed that there was some obligation to carry out research with embryos, which I do not either. I would argue that "nothing is lost"—to turn Outka's argument on its head—by not doing the research at all (as I explained earlier).

## CONCLUSION

I conclude with a few observations on the regulation of stem cell research. For at least three decades, the strategy of choice for dealing with morally controversial scientific initiatives which have strong scientific support has been to establish commissions, which propose some limits and then turn the problem over to a regulatory approach. The National Academy of Sciences on stem cell research put together a commission that set forth a number of regulatory ideas (hoping, it appears, to avoid a similar government move), and the state of California as well as some academic research centers have set standards for carrying out the research.[29] But we should not expect commissions and regulations to stop the research. Their purpose is to reduce anxieties about it and to curtail evident abuses. It would be a miracle if any ardent research opponents were appointed members of those commissions or asked to help write the regulations. The aim of the commissions is, after all, to facilitate the research—to make sure it goes forward—but in ways that keep hostile legislators and a worried public at bay.[30] That's the American way, and it well serves those ends, even if at times we pay an ethical price for it. The most important price is that it allows us to keep going with the research but salves our conscience in the process, and it is hardly noticed.

I end my paper with one sentence. The moral status of early embryos is weak and uncertain, but not nearly as weak as the moral status of research cloning.

*Notes*

1. See Daniel Callahan, Abortion: Law, Choice And Morality (1970).

2. See Exec. Order No. 13,505, 74 Fed. Reg. 10,667 (Mar. 9, 2009); Sheryl Gay Stolberg, *New Stem Cell Policy To Leave Thorniest Issue to Congress*, N.Y. Times, Mar. 9, 2009, at Al; David Stout & Gardiner Harris, *Obama Reversing Stem Cell Limits Imposed by Bush*, N.Y. Times, Mar. 7, 2009, at Al, available at http://www.nytimes.com/2009/03/07/us/politics/07stem.html.

3. For a listing of state funding, see James W. Fossett, *Beyond the Low-Hanging Fruit: Stem Cell Research Policy in an Obama Administration*, 9 Yale J. Health Policy & Ethics 523 (2009).

4. *See* Daniel Callahan, What Price Better Health?: Hazards of the Research Imperative (2003).

5. National Institutes of Health, Research Portfolio Online Reporting Tool (RePORT), Estimates of Funding for Various Research, Condition and Disease Categories (RCDC), http://report.nih.gov/rcdc/categories (last visited Apr. 30, 2009).

6. Nicholas Wade, *Some Scientists See Shift in Stem Cell Hopes*, N.Y. Times, Aug. 14, 2006, at A18.

7. Felix Montes & Roy L. Johnson, *The New Stale of Illiteracy in San Antonio and the Nation*, Intercultural Dev. Res. Ass'n Newsl., April 2005, *available at* http://www.idra.org/IDRA_Newsletter/April_2005_Self__Renewing_Schools_Reading_and_Liter    acy/The_New_State_of_Illiteracy_in_San_Antonio_and_in_the_Nation.

8. James A. Thomson et al., *Embryonic Stem Cell Lines Derived from Human Blastocysts*, 282 Science 1145 (1998).

9. Elizabeth Brenner Drew, *The Health Syndicate: Washington's Noble Conspirators*, Atlantic Monthly, Dec. 1967, at 75.

10. *See generally* Alliance for Aging Research, Embryonic Stem Cell Research To Save the Lives of Millions, Spring 2001, http://www.agingresearch.org/content/article/detail/917 (outlining hopes for future stem cell technologies).

11. *See* T. Hviid Nielsen, *10 Years of Stem Cells: What Happened to the Stem Cells?*, 34 J. Med. Ethics 852, 853 2008).

12. *See* Rick Weiss, *Nobel (Laureates Back Stem Cell Research*, Wash. Post, Feb. 22, 2001, at A2.

13. Tinker Ready,...*and ES Cell Strategy,* 7 Nature Med. 518, 518 (2001) (describing the open letter from college presidents to Health and Human Services Secretary Tommy Thompson).

14. John M. Broder & Andrew Pollack, *Californians To Vote on Spending $3 Billion for Stem Cell Research,* N.Y. Times, Sept. 20, 2004, at A23.

15. For an example of this rhetoric, see Robert Kuttner, *When We Trust Science to Religion,* San Diego Union-Trib., Dec. 9,2001, at G3.

16. Sheryl Gay Stolberg, *The Biotech Death of Jesse Gelsinger,* N.Y. Times, Nov. 28, 1999, § 6 (Magazine), at 137.

17. Gail Collins, *Public Interests; A Shot in the Dark,* N.Y. Times, June 30, 2000, at A25.

18. Gretchen Vogel, *Korean Team Speeds Up Creation of Cloned Human Cells,* 309 Science 1096 (2005).

19. Alan Boyle, *Stem Cell Pioneer Does a Reality Check: James Thomson Reflects on Science and Morality,* MSNBC.com, June 25, 2005, http://www.msnbc.msn.com/id/8303756.

20. *Ibid.*

21. *Ibid.*

22. Andrew Pollack, *Milestone in Research in Stem Cells,* N.Y. Times, Jan. 23, 2009, at Bl.

23. Office of the Sec'y, Dep't of Health, Educ, & Welfare, Protection of Human Subjects: HEW Support of In Vitro Fertilization and Embryo Transfer: Report of the Ethics Advisory Board, 44 Fed. Reg. 35,033, at 35,056 (June 18, 1979).

24. Nat'l Inst of Health, Report of the Human Embryo Research Panel, at x (1994), *available at* http://bioethics.georgetown.edu/pcbe/reports/past_commissions/human_ embryo_vol_1.pdf.

25. Nat'l Bioethics Advisory Comm'n, Ethical Issues in Human Stem Cell Research, at ii (1999), *available at* http://bioethics.georgetown.edu/nbac/stemcell.pdf.

26. *The American Heritage Dictionary of the English Language* 1107 (1st ed. 1969).

27. *See* Repro-Gen Ethics and the Future of Gender (Frida Simonstein ed., forthcoming June 2009).

28. Gretchen Vogel, *Embryo-Free Techniques Gain Momentum,* 309 Science 240 (2005).

29. *See* Comm. on Guidelines for Human Embryonic Stem Cell Research, Nat'l Research Council, Guidelines for Human Embryonic Stem Cell Research (2005), *available at* http:// www.nap.edu/openbook.php?isbn=0309096537.

30. John H. Evans, Playing God? Human Genetic Engineering and the Rationalization of Public Bioethical Debate (2002).

# HEALTH TECHNOLOGY ASSESSMENT
# IMPLEMENTATION: THE POLITICS OF ETHICS

The ethical considerations and problems of health technology assessment (HTA) can roughly be put in 2 categories, one of which can be called interior and the other exterior. By "interior," I mean that part of HTA that focuses on the methodologies used by HTA to collect and assess data, which have been called the methodological standards. I will not comment on those issues, important though they are. Instead, I will be concerned with what I call the "exterior" ethical issues, by which I mean those that arise in the move from data collection and the judgment of the researchers to their dissemination and use in the medical community and, beyond that, to the public as well.

Aristotle contended that ethics is a branch of politics. I want to contend that the professional and public acceptance of HTA depends upon the ethical acceptability of its recommendations. But its acceptability in that respect cannot be separated from the politics and values of the health care system of which it is a part.

As I will try to show, the debate about, and often resistance to, HTA in the United States rests on a number of ethical values and principles. At bottom, that debate, which can look like nothing more than politics—understood narrowly as a clash of interest groups vying for dominance—is an ethical debate and one that has to be resolved at that level. I will use the major 2009 American debate on mammography screening for breast cancer as a starting point to make clear the intertwining of ethics and politics. I will then move on to an examination of HTA more broadly, aiming to understand the likely political difficulties it will encounter in the future as the combination of aging societies and more expensive medical technologies lead it into ever more troubled waters. My focus will be on the United States, not simply because I know its health care system best but because the politics of HTA has been particularly vexed, offering a cautionary tale for other countries so far blessed with more coherent health care systems.

## THE RESEARCH RECOMMENDATION AND ITS CRITICISMS

In 2009, The US Preventive Services Task Force (PSTF) recommended that mammography for women under the age of 50 years should not be routinely prescribed and that, for women between that age and 74 years, screening was best done only every 2 years.[1] For women under the age of 50 years, individual decisions should be made based on the patient's history and values. Not only is there a reduced risk of breast cancer for women under 50 years, the task force held, but there can also be psychological problems, false-positive findings, and the harms of unnecessary treatment and radiation exposure. At no point do the recommendations mention costs as a consideration.

The recommendations were promptly, publicly, and widely attacked by various medical interest groups (The American Cancer Society, The American College of Radiology, and the National Cancer Institute); by breast cancer survivors; and by patient advocacy groups. They were said to be excessive, a serious threat to the lives of women under 50 years. The criticisms were quickly taken up and amplified by politically conservative groups as a dangerous incursion of government into the doctor-patient relationship and as an opening salvo in rationing care. The fact that the recommendations took place in the midst of the American health reform debate, part of which encompassed HTA, served to amplify the furor. Nonetheless, despite some gestures in that direction, there were no serious criticisms of the research methodology, and the PSTF has a solid reputation for the quality of its research. Even so, the attack evoked a defensive response from the Obama administration, with Secretary of the Department of Health and Human Resources, Kathleen Sibelius, emphasizing that in the end screening decisions should be left up to doctors and their patients, effectively marginalizing the PSTF recommendations.

## HISTORICAL RESISTANCE TO HTA

HTA has had a troubled history in the United States, of which the mammography struggle is just a recent instance. But it has also had a peculiar kind of history.

HTA, and even cost-benefit studies, together with practice guidelines based on them, have been numerous over the years within some federal agencies, medical specialty groups, and private industry. The state of Washington, for instance, quietly runs an HTA program, encompassing evidence of treatment effectiveness, safety, and comparative effectiveness research (CER).[2]

When HTA is raised to the federal level, however, that is a disconcertingly different story. The US Medicare program for the elderly has been forbidden since its initiation in 1965 from using cost-benefit research (CBR) to make benefit decisions. "Reasonable and necessary," an inherently vague concept, is the only acceptable standard. Decades of complaints by Medicare administrators about this policy have had no effect. A Center for Health Care Technology was established in 1978 and then summarily killed in 1981 because of complaints by the American Medical Association and the Health Industry Manufacturers Association.[3] A productive Office of Technology Assessment (but only in part focused on medical technologies), established in 1972 by Congress, lost its funding in 1995. The work of the Agency for Health Care Research and Quality, established in 1985, and responsible for HTA, had its mission seriously curtailed in great part because of complaints by back surgeons about an agency decision in favor of a nonsurgical approach.

That history of resistance, and often hostility, to HTA was prominently on display in the health care reform debate. In its run up to the final legislation, the Obama administration included in a package of measures designed to deal with the financial recession $1.1 billion for CER. That money was then folded into the reform legislation but with the firm stipulation that the research findings could not be used to establish practice guidelines or even to make recommendations. The hand of industry was heavy.[4] While CER can be valuable, that prohibition effectively neutered it as a direct means of cost control, one of the principal aims of the reform bill. Along the way to the reform bill, moreover, the dread word "rationing" was rhetorically treated as the logical outcome of HTA, with even CER as some of the grease on the slippery slope, and all the worse because faceless government bureaucrats would do the dirty work. The dread specter of an American National Institute for Health and Clinical Excellence (NICE) agency wielding quality-adjusted life years (QALYs) was advanced as the means of rationing. Even so, hardly anyone denied that CER could be of some value; it just has to be kept on a tight leash.

## ETHICS AND POLITICS

At first glance, the troubled history of HTA can appear to be nothing other than a display of the political power of the various interest groups long dominant in

American medicine and health care: the medical profession, various industry groups, and conservative antigovernment political forces. But what is striking about their politics is that its arguments and rhetoric invoke ethical principles as their foundation. Industry resistance to HTA stems from a long-standing fear of government price controls and invokes market freedom as its ethical principle (a freedom necessary for democratic freedom). The resistance of some physician groups is based on the ancient belief that the highest goal of medicine is individual health. They believe that ethical goal will be lost with the probabilistic studies endemic to CER, focused on group data and not on individual patients in all their variety ("every patient is different"). The closely related ethical value of the doctor-patient relationship, traditionally referred to by the American Medical Association as the "sacred doctor-patient relation-ship," is seen as a high wall to keep out the government from bureaucratically interfering with it.

The comparative effectiveness work of the reform legislation centers on the creation of a public–private initiative called the Patient-Centered Outcomes Research Institute. It will have a board of directors of 21 persons, drawn from a mix of representatives of special interests and of 2 government health agen-cies. The fight over this institute was almost epic in its complexity and ferocity. As John Iglehart, an astute observer of the health care scene and the founding editor of *Health Affairs*, wrote, the survival of the institute concept "illustrates how Congress's majority ultimately prevailed over Republican rhetoric about a 'government takeover' and rationing of health care. On another level, it's a story of how the Democrats succeeded only after making a series of accommodations with private interests."[5]

At bottom, the political struggle about CER comes down to an ethical clash of market-oriented individualist values, with the ethical value of freedom at its core, and a common good/solidarity set of ethical values. Unless I am mistaken about HTA in other developed countries, my impression is that the European health care's ethical foundation in the value of solidarity has made it easier to introduce both CER and CBR. America's congenital individualism, as well as the active role played by physicians, industry groups, and patient advocacy groups, has made it much harder in the United States.

Yet, if the much-noted American "exceptionalism" is on display in the CER debate, why do I call it a cautionary tale for other countries, so far blessed with a greater willingness to embrace HTA? First of all, I believe the growing prob-lem of cost escalation in every developed country, intensified as the proportion of elderly continues to grow and the dependency ratio of workers to retirees worsens, will put more and more pressure on health care systems to drastically control costs.

Second, the steady stream of new and improved medical technologies will intensify the cost problem. As the American Congressional Budget Office noted in a 2008 report, "examples of new treatments for which long-term savings have been clearly demonstrated are few...improvement in medical care that decreases mortality...paradoxically increase overall spending on health care because surviving patients live longer and therefore use health services for more years."[6] Most recent medical progress has served up not cures of chronic disease but the ability to keep those with such diseases alive longer and more expensively.

Third, while there are already complaints and problems with expensive pharmaceuticals for the treatment of cancer—$50,000 to $100,000 for some with only a small increase in life expectancy—it is reasonable to anticipate that sooner or later, some drugs will come along for some major cancer (e.g., breast cancer) that for a similarly high price will increase life expectancies for years and not just months. Think of it as the economic doomsday drug. Every woman with the disease would clamor for it, and no agency, public or private, would want to provide it. At a somewhat lower level of economic horror, the much touted advent of personalized genetic medicine has been hailed as a major new medical frontier, but there is every expectation that it will be expensive.

In short, I would expect that at present, and even with the use of QALYs, very few technologies and treatments will fall into the category of intolerable costs for minimum benefits, much less intolerable costs for even larger benefits. NICE issues negative judgments on only somewhere between 10% and 13% of the technologies submitted for review.[7] That situation is likely to change as the technologies get more effective and, with a growing elderly population, there are proportionately more people on whom to use them. HTA decisions against treatments will, correspondingly, get to be more common, more difficult, and more controversial. Then other countries, relatively quiescent so far, will run the risk, even the likelihood, of a revolt by physicians, industry, and the public.

## RESPONDING TO THE ETHICAL AND POLITICAL PROBLEMS

It is not clear to what extent the PSTF anticipated the hostility of the many groups that spoke out against its recommendations, much less the way those critics made their criticisms public by immediately going to the media. It was not a quiet debate among researchers over differences to be resolved politely in professional journals. The critics made sure of that.

What lessons can be learned from that event, which has some parallels in reactions to NICE decisions in the United Kingdom? I think of that problem in terms of a kind of preventive medicine. The obvious starting point is that the science behind the research, at what I earlier called the "interior" category, must be solid and in particular untainted by outside interested parties, whether government officials, industry concerns, and patient groups. The research process, that is, must be as transparent as possible.

So far as possible, the major stakeholders in the research outcomes and recommendations should have a role as commentators at the beginning, the middle, and the end of the research process. But does that suggestion not contradict my first recommendation of keeping the research process untainted by interested parties? Not if it is done carefully. Their opinions and ideas should be welcomed and their interests put on the table, while at the same time, making clear that the researchers must be ruled in the end by the ethic of scientific research, which has its own professional rules. If that exchange is done well, and in a collegial way, it should be possible to anticipate the responses of those interest groups when the findings and recommendations are made public.

The recommendations themselves require the greatest care. I believe there is a general public belief that HTA comes to simple yes-or-no judgments: things work, or they do not. The reality, of course, is that of probabilistic judgments, far more in the gray area than black or white. The PSTF recommendations do not say "do not screen under 50." Bearing in mind a variety of adverse hazards for women 40 to 49 years, they say "there is moderate certainty that the net benefit is small."

No numbers are attached to the "moderate certainty" judgment, just as there are no numbers provided for the possible adverse events (e.g., false-positive results leading to biopsies, anxiety, and other stresses). In short, a judgment was made, an all-things-considered, on-balance judgment. It is doubtful that much more precision could have been brought to the study, and it is obvious (as some critics loudly noted) that some otherwise low-risk women from 40 to 49 years not screened would develop breast cancer and be at risk of death. The same could be said of routine screening of women 30 to 39 years. Just as the recommendations were coming out, a young colleague of mine told me about a 20-year-old friend of hers who believed she detected lumps in her breast. But she could not at first persuade her university doctors to perform a mammography. It was, they said, highly improbable that she could at her age have breast cancer. Indeed so, but they did screen anyway because she was obviously anxious, and she did have cancer. Stories like that get around.

I might add that, if the physician of a woman at, say, age 35 years, should for reasons of family history or other considerations decide to screen her, he could probably provide no hard risk data either if his patient were skeptical. In short, there will almost always be uncertainty, conflicting judgments even among those who agree on the evidence, and even more opportunities for doubt and contro-versy when the recommendations go out to a public, including physicians look-ing for certainty and not carefully formulated, prudential judgments. The pitfalls of making judgments are many, and at least in the American context, there are enough alleged experts around ready to jump on HTA conclusions.

In a 2007 work written for the Biotechnology Industry Organization, *The Complexities of Comparative Effectiveness*, Dr. Ted Buckley worked his way through an intimidating long list of those complexities: for instance, the lack of a standard definition of just what CER is, a history of health care providers and patients who do not pay attention to relevant information anyway, population-based studies not pertinent to individual patient needs, and so on.[8] His aim, he says, is simply "edu-cation" about the complexities, but by the end of the work, it would seem that CER is so mired in that jungle of complexity that only fools would even attempt it. He is not wrong about the complexities, but they seem no worse than in other sectors of human life: predictions about climate change, the best foreign policy for dealing with China, assessing the hazards of nuclear reactors in one's neighborhood, and offshore drilling. That is just the way modern life is. I am not certain I would ask Dr. Buckley whether it is safe to get out of bed in the morning.

Most of everything I have said so far points in one direction, that of the need for much improved public and professional education. Not only is that necessary for the sake of scientific literacy about HTA but all the more so to alert doctors and the public about the way various interest groups can sometimes shape data to their own ends or to debunk even the most careful studies. I would particularly single out the importance of educating the media as well. Not only is it rare for the public to read, or readily understand, complex scientific findings, but many physicians (at least in my own experience) are also less than assiduous in keeping up with the medical literature. They are also as likely to be alerted to new studies and data by the media as the general public.

My guess, for instance, is that many physicians first learned about the mam-mography debate from the extensive news coverage, not from picking it up directly from the *Annals of Internal Medicine* where it was published. For the most part, the reporting was balanced and careful but dealt little with its meth-odology or the nuance of its recommendations. And it did not direct attention as much as it might have to the self-interest of some of the medical and professional groups that were the most critical. Workshops and special conferences for the media about HTA would be most fruitful. I doubt there is more than a handful of American reporters and medical writers who could be said to be experts on the subject. If and when some truly momentous struggle breaks out over an HTA study and recommendation, the reporting of it in the media is likely to be of the highest importance.

## PERENNIAL PROBLEMS

Three problems are likely to dog the footsteps of HTA: prevention studies, the treatment of statistical outliers, and HTA and the role of the physician (the art and science of medicine).

The mammography screening recommendation is a type of study whose findings will often be controversial. In essence, how many people is it worth screening in order to find a comparative few who will benefit from treatment? As the portion of beneficiaries declines, for instance, from 60% to 50% all the way down to 1%, at what point does it make no economic sense to carry out the screening? QALYs analysis can in principle answer that question, but inevitably, there would be some denied screening whose life might have been saved; and in this social media era, their names are likely to be known.

At least in the mammography case, it could be shown that the screening could itself have adverse effects, allowing a tradeoff between different kinds of health risks and benefits. Screening procedures ruled out at some level solely on economic grounds would have no such redeeming virtues. In the case of cost alone, a recommendation not to screen beyond a certain point would simply look cold and cruel, however valid the research design. The only way to lessen the negative public impact would be to enhance the efforts suggested above: to ensure that the likely affected interest groups were fully aware of the ongoing research, and with a strong consultative role from beginning to end, and that the media were signaled in advance what the recommendations would likely be. Avoid surprises.

There is a phrase in the competitive golfing world about tournament players who do not "make the cut." By that phrase, it is meant that if, early in a tournament, a golfer does not achieve a minimum score, he or she will not be allowed to continue further. They are just out of the tournament altogether. Some HTA recommendations will mean that, for economic or other reasons, some patients will not be eligible for a particular treatment; they will not "make the cut." The ethical dilemma of considering their fate is of the worst kind. They are not responsible for the fact that their disease, or their status with it, is not their fault. We cannot say to them, "why did you choose to have this disease?" Getting it was their bad luck. They are losers in the lottery for treatment, the statistical outliers.

They will put HTA to its most severe test. To pass this test, HTA must have a secure scientific and public reputation, legislators and the public must understand the resource scarcity that makes such outcomes necessary, and the recommendations must not be presented as an impersonal bureaucratic decision but as the resolution of an unpleasant and difficult moral dilemma. If at all possible, efforts to enlist industry support for those outliers should be solicited. Their prices for drugs or devices will be part of the problem, and they can be considered a source of the moral dilemma, one that is as likely to give them a public black eye as HTA. They would be wise; it should be expressly pointed out to them to do what they can to relieve the economic burden leading to such a decision. But that will not always be feasible, in which case the public standing and integrity of the HTA agency will be the critical variable.

It has long been understood within the profession that medicine properly understood is both science and art. The science comes from the broad generalizations about the human body made possible by scientific research, whether biological or HTA. The art comes from an understanding that patients are different, that experience and judgment come into play in trying to simultaneously bring those skills together with the scientific knowledge in the treatment of individual patients. The good physician is understood to be one who knows how to do that and knows it can be difficult on occasion.

Yet, it is also known that some physicians are too much swayed by their limited experience, by the practices of their neighboring colleagues, or simply by the fact that they do not work hard to keep their scientific knowledge up to date. The common but seemingly counterintuitive advice that a patient might do better with a young, newly minted physician filled with the latest information than a much older, more experienced one reflects that background perception, reflecting a certain skepticism about physician judgment. The fact that many physicians have long been notorious for not acting on well-known and published HTA findings bears out that skepticism. I have a physician who is much loved, sensitive to me as a person, and thought well of professionally. But I long ago discovered how awkward it is for me to ask him, concerning some of my medical conditions, if he has read this or that journal article on recent evidence of diagnostic or treatment strategies. Too often, he has not and is a bit sheepish about that. Nonetheless, he has so many other physician virtues that I have not sought a change.

In other words, I am sympathetic to physician worries that HTA will impose rigid guidelines on their behavior or limit what they can, in their best judgment, prescribe for their patients. Even so, too much sympathy would be a mistake given how hard it is to get many physicians to take evidence seriously and change their practice habits accordingly. The refusal by our Congress to allow the use of CER to establish practice guidelines or even to make recommendations seemed to me and many others to have been a huge mistake, which many critics are even now working to change, however difficult that may be, and similar efforts are underway with cost-benefit analysis.[9] The Secretary of the Department of Health and Human Services should not, as noted above, have given in to the interest groups that objected to the mammography recommendations, undercutting a reputable agency that works under her authority in her own department and particularly when those recommendations make clear that they could be overridden in individual cases.

I can offer no clear advice on the best way to get physicians to take seriously HTA evidence and act upon recommendations. A strictly regulatory approach aiming to micromanage physicians would not only put aside the important tradition of deference to physician judgment in treating their patients but also would bring HTA into disrepute because of its insensitivity to patient differences. Yet, bland recommendations will not do too much good either. I believe the PSTF has a reasonable way of dealing with that kind of dilemma. In making use of a grading system for its recommendations—ranging from "A" for services where there is a "high certainty that net benefit is substantial" through "D," a recommendation against the service—it makes clear its own standards and the weight of potential pressure behind them. In the case of its mammography recommendations, it gives them a grade of "C," which is a recommendation "against routinely providing the service."

That kind of recommendation leaves considerable room for physician judgment with individual patients, but it also deals effectively with a common criticism of HTA that it supplies only a "one-size-for-all" judgment. Its "A" grade might be said to do that, but it can be applied only when the evidence is overwhelming. When that is the case, its recommendations can legitimately be used to put considerable pressure on physicians, socially as well as professionally. If I am sometimes embarrassed to cite my Internet findings to my doctor, I would have no objection to an HTA agency using that same resource to tell physicians how they might, all things considered, make use of evidence in their treatment patterns. And we, their patients, can be listening in.


## THE POLITICS OF ETHICS

I have tried in this article to interpret the meaning of the mammography debate in the United States in terms of the interplay of ethics and politics. Ethics as a long-established academic discipline has historically sought to remove itself from the political arena, not out of distaste for it but instead to see if some enduring moral values, principles, rules, and virtues can be fashioned that will help us shape our own lives as individuals and our social relationships with others. One important way to pursue that goal is to examine the way people actually live their lives, the way they articulate their values, and the implicit and explicit moral rules common in their society and its subgroups. The political arena is one place to focus attention and, in the mammography case, the medical arena as well.

As the American health care debate has made clear, there is a fundamental split between those for whom the ethical values of freedom and individual choice are paramount and those for whom the collective common good is most important. In the context of health care, the former set of values often draws heavily on some ancient medical values, notably the primacy of the individual doctor-patient relationship and not the collective health of the public. The common good approach, by contrast, often articulated in the language of solidarity in European countries, stresses the mutual interdependence of human beings, their common neediness in the face of illness, and the obligation to support each other in paying for health care. Layered on top of those ethical struggles is a fierce debate about the role of government. One side, in the tradition of Thomas Jefferson, is hostility to a strong government role, not only in health care but most other areas of American life (save for national defense); the other side, invoking justice, looks to government to facilitate our obligations to others in time of need. The market, on the other side, is seen as the main economic vehicle for the expression of choice, with as little government interference as possible.

In the end, this political/ideological/ethical struggle comes down to a fundamental clash of different visions of how to live our individual and collective lives. American HTA must do its work in that vexing context. If HTA is envisioned in an ethically minimalist way, doing nothing but collecting and assessing data but passing no judgment on its clinical or other uses, it can pass muster with those worried about judgments making use of that data to interfere with the commercial drug and device industries or the private doctor–patient relationship. The political clout of those interests accounted for the limits placed on government-sponsored CER. But effective HTA, I believe, must be used to establish clinical guidelines, allow for assessments of opportunity costs among competing technologies, and have an important place in health care budgeting. But then, I am on the side of a solidarity-based, government-regulated, universal access health care system, and HTA at its strongest best fits into that kind of system.

The utility of ethics, and its best contribution, comes when it is possible to introduce ethical principles and rules into a context that is still open to different perspectives and in need of some guidance. The trouble comes when there are 2 or more competitive value systems, each of which has been fashioned and polished by its adherents into a coherent, tight system. The history of moral theories— for instance, utilitarianism versus duty-oriented systems—is that their adherents have worked on them and turned them into (in their eyes) plausible and internally consistent theories, not readily admitting of compromise. The ideological and political struggle over health care in the United States is a clash between such theories. Understood in that way, one could say that the problem is not a lack of ethics but a clash of incompatible theories that each blends ethical values and political values together in a way not easily open to moderation or compromise.

The result in the United States is, in effect, both an ethical and a political stalemate, one marked by intransigence on both sides among politicians as well as the general public. As I write this in the spring of 2011, it is simply impossible even to guess how the stalemate will be broken and a compromise brought about. The field of ethics has itself over the centuries displayed analogous stalemates, many of them resolved by the entrance of new theories. No such opening is now apparent in the health care reform struggle nor in the deployment of HTA. One side welcomes it and will push to strengthen it, moving toward its use in shaping policy and influencing physician behavior. The other side sees it as a danger to be combated and its impact nullified or minimized. A problem of that kind cannot be solved by the invocation of ethics. It is a clash of ethics that is itself at the core of the problem. The fate of HTA is thus up in the air, along with the rest of American health care reform.

## References

1. US Services Task Force. Screening for breast cancer: U.S. Preventive Services Task Force Recommendation Statement. Ann Intern Med. 2009;151:716–26.
2. Fox J. Medicare should, but cannot consider cost: legal impediments to a sound policy. Buffalo Law Rev. 2005;53:577–633.
3. Callahan D. Taming the Beloved Beast: How Medical Technology Costs Are Destroying Our Health Care System. Princeton: Princeton University Press; 2009. p l22–124.
4. Selker HP, Wood AJ. Industry influence on comparative effectiveness research funded through health care reform. N Engl J Med. 2009;361(27):2595–2597.
5. Iglehart JK. The political fight over comparative effectiveness research. Health Aff. 2010;29:1777–1782.
6. Congressional Budget Office. Technological Change and the Growth of Health Care Spending. Washington, DC: Congressional Budget Office; 2008.
7. Clement FM, Harris A, Li JJ, Yong K, Lee KM, Manns BJ. Using effectiveness and cost-effectiveness to make drug coverage decisions: a comparison of Britain, Australia, and Canada. JAMA. 2009;302(13):1437–1443.
8. Buckley T. The Complexities of Comparative Effectiveness. Washington, DC: Biotechnology Industry Organization; 2007.
9. Garber AM, Sox HC. The role of costs in comparative effectiveness research. Health Aff. 2010;29:1805–1811.

# BIOETHICS AND FATHERHOOD

## I. INTRODUCTION

For most of the rest of our culture, the twin issues of the meaning of masculinity (or maleness, depending on your tastes), and the significance of fatherhood are well-developed topics of public discussion. Whether as a response to feminism, on the one hand, or to independent uncertainties about what it means to be a male, on the other, the question of masculinity attracts considerable attention. While fatherhood was not exactly a neglected topic in years past, there seems little doubt that the nasty phenomena of more and more single-parent families, mainly headed by females, and a growing number of absent and neglectful fathers, has given the issue a fresh urgency. What does it mean to be a father? What is the importance of the father for the nurturing of children? What can be done to encourage and assist more responsible fatherhood? What is the relationship between fatherhood and masculinity?

These are interesting and important questions, and timely as well. One would, however, never guess that from reading the literature of bioethics. For whatever reason, that literature, when it focuses on gender at all, is almost exclusively interested in women. And when it focuses on parenthood, it almost exclusively focuses on motherhood. While the general topics of reproductive choices and artificial means of reproduction have had a central place in bioethics, the literature and debate have usually centered on women's choices or women's role in such things as surrogate motherhood and *in vitro* fertilization. Fathers and fatherhood are just absent from the discussion altogether.

The absence of fatherhood in the debate is puzzling, especially since the topic of artificial means of reproduction is a central one in the field. My surmise is that, because those means of reproduction depend so heavily upon anonymous male sperm donations, and since such donations are rarely questioned for their moral propriety, there has been no need or place to talk about fathers. They just don't really count in that brave new world of reproduction. I will return later to that topic. Of more general importance is whether fatherhood can be given a fresh look and a reinvigorated role in bioethics.

At the heart of the problem and future of parenthood, and thus of the most basic and indispensable kind of human nurturing, is a *relationship*, of men, women, and children bound together. Professionals seem to have lost a sense of and feel for that relationship—of the way men, women, and children need and best flourish in the company of the other. Instead, professionals have done conceptually what society has been doing legally and socially—treating men, women, and children as separate and distinguishable, with their own needs and rights. Thus we now speak easily of women's rights, and children's rights, and (hardly surprising, even if amusing) we have seen the growth of a men's rights movement. Doubtless there are some good reasons for this fragmenting development, the most important being the way earlier generations were prone to stack the family relationship, and its ground rules, too heavily in favor of men; or, where children were concerned, to treat them too much as the property of their parents, not as persons in their own rights.

But it is time for some reintegration. The fragmentation is, unless corrected in the long run, going to be harmful for men, women, and children, both individually and in their relationship. A revived and reinvigorated place for fathers and the institution of fatherhood is as good a place as any to begin. I want to develop three points: (1) biological fatherhood carries with it permanent and nondispensable duties; (2) the rapid and widespread acceptance of artificial insemination donors was much too thoughtless and casual, but for just that reason symbolic of the devaluation of fatherhood; and (3) feminism as a movement has hurt both men and children, but also women, by its tendency to substantively displace fathers from a central role in the making of procreation decisions.

## II. THE DUTIES OF FATHERHOOD

I begin here with the most simple and primitive of moral axioms, rarely articulated as such but as undeniable as anything can possibly be in ethics. The axiom is this: Human beings bear a moral responsibility for those voluntary acts that have an impact on the lives of others; they are morally accountable for such acts. I will not discuss the many nuances and problems that this axiom raises: what counts as "voluntary," how great must be the impact upon others, and which effects of actions on others are morally more or less important.

In the case of biological fatherhood those nuances will not ordinarily be of great importance. From this moral axiom I will argue that given the obvious importance of procreation in bringing human life into existence, fathers have a significant moral responsibility for the children they voluntarily procreate. What human action could be more important than that which creates new life, the burden of which the newly born person must live with for the rest of his or her life? What causal connection could be more direct than biological procreation, without which human existence would not be possible? A father can hardly be held wholly responsible for *what* a child becomes—much will depend upon circumstances—but a father can be held responsible with the mother for the fact the child comes to be at all.

One philosopher has advanced the notion that our only serious moral obligations are those we voluntarily impose upon ourselves, as in specific contracts.[1] There cannot be, she says, involuntary obligations. This is not the place to debate the full implications of such a theory—which must systematically close its eyes to what it means to live in a community with other people—but it is pertinent to make a single point. Unless a male is utterly naive about the facts of procreation, to engage in voluntary sexual intercourse is to be responsible for what happens as a result. To enter into a contract with another is, at the least, to undertake a voluntary activity with a known likely outcome. Sexual intercourse for an informed male is fairly close to that, so even on a contract theory of moral obligation, intercourse shares many critical features with a contract. Society, curiously, seems to have been faster in establishing the moral and causal links between drinking and driving than between sexual activity and pregnancy. But that may be because society prefers to think that accidental, unwanted pregnancies come more from contraceptive ignorance and failure than from the sexual activities that require them; the former is a more comforting thought to sustain the sexual revolution.

From my moral axiom, therefore, and from what we know about the biology of human procreation, I believe there is no serious way of denying the moral seriousness of biological fatherhood and the existence of moral duties that follow from it. The most important moral statement might be this: Once a father, always a father. Because the relationship is biological rather than contractual, the natural bond cannot be abrogated or put aside. I conclude, that just as society cannot put aside the biological bond, so neither ought it put aside the moral bond, the set of obligations that go with that biological bond. If there are to be moral duties at all, then the biological bond is as fundamental and unavoidable as any that can be imagined.[2] Does this mean that each and every father has a full set of moral obligations toward the children he procreates? My answer is yes—unless he is mentally or financially incompetent to discharge those duties. To treat the matter otherwise is to assume that fatherhood *is* some kind of contractual relationship, one that can be set aside by some choice on the part of the father, or the mother and father together, or on the part of the state. This position does not preclude allowing one person to adopt the child of another, to play the role of father with a legal sanction to do so. This arrangement, however, is legitimate only when there are serious obstacles standing in the way of the biological father playing that role himself. Even then, however, he remains the biological father, and should the alternative arrangements for the child fail, he is once again responsible, and responsible whether he likes it or not, accepts it or not. The obligation stems from his original, irreversible act of procreation; so too is his moral obligation irreversible.

Imagine the following scenario. A father has, through the assorted legal ways society allows fathers to turn over their parental authority to another, legally ceased to act as a father and someone else is caring for the child. But imagine that the other person fails to adequately act as a father; fails, that is, to properly care for and nurture the child. The child then returns to the father and says: "You are still my father biologically; because of you I exist in this world. I need your help and you are obliged to give it to me." I have never been able to imagine even *one* moral reason why a father in that circumstance could disclaim responsibility, and disclaim it if, even in principle, there was someone else available who could take care of the child. A father is a father is a father.

## III. FATHERHOOD AND ARTIFICIAL INSEMINATION

I find it remarkable that, with hardly any public debate at all, the practice—indeed, institution—of artificial insemination by an anonymous male donor so easily slipped in. What could society have been thinking about? In this section I will argue that it is fundamentally wrong and should have no place in a civilized, much less a supposedly liberal society. It is wrong for just the reasons I have sketched in Section II about the moral obligations that go with fatherhood. A sperm donor whose sperm is successfully used to fertilize an ovum, which ovum proceeds through the usual phases of gestation, is a *father*. Nothing more, nothing less. He is as much a father biologically as the known sperm inseminator in a standard heterosexual relationship and sexual intercourse.

If he is thereby a biological father, he has all the duties of any other biological father. It is morally irrelevant that (1) the donor does not want to act as a father, (2) those who collect his sperm as medical brokers do not want him to act as a father, (3) the woman whose ovum he is fertilizing does not want him to act as a father, and (4) society is prepared to excuse him from the obligations of acting as a father. Fatherhood, because it is a biological condition, cannot be abrogated by personal desires or legal decisions. Nor can the moral obligations be abrogated either, unless there are reasons why they *cannot* be discharged, not simply that no one wants them to be discharged. Just as a "surrogate mother" is not a "surrogate" at all but a perfectly real and conventional biological mother, so also is a sperm donor whose sperm results in a child a perfectly real and conventional biological father.

Why was it decided to set all that aside? Why was it deemed acceptable for males to become fathers by becoming sperm donors but then to relieve them *totally* of all responsibility of being fathers, leaving this new father ignorant of who his child is and the child ignorant of who the father is? I was not present at that great cultural moment, but two reasons seem to have been paramount.

First, it was introduced under medical auspices and given a medical legitimation. Artificial insemination by a donor ("AID"), one author wrote, is "medically indicated in instances of the man's sterility, possible hereditary disease, rhesus incompatibility, or in most cases of oligospermia."[3] "Medically indicated?" But it does not cure anyone's disease—not some other would-be father who is sterile, or the woman who receives the sperm who is perfectly capable of motherhood without donated sperm. What is cured, so to speak, is a couple's desire to have a child; but medicine does not ordinarily treat relational problems (save in psychotherapy), so there is no reason to call the matter medical at all. Moreover, of course, since artificial insemination only requires a single syringe, inserted in a well-known place, there is nothing "medical" even about the procedure.

As Daniel Wikler has nicely pointed out, the professional dominance of doctors in the history of AID is a perfect case of the medicalization of a nonmedical act, and the establishment of a medical monopoly and legitimization as a result.[4] Just how far this medicalization has gone can be seen by the very language used to describe the procedure: "[Artificial Insemination] is of two basic types: homologous, when the semen is obtained from the husband (AIH); and heterologous, when the semen is acquired from a donor (AID)."[5] I wonder how many males, working pleasurably to produce some sperm, understood themselves to be engaged in a heterologous activity? There is very little that medical science cannot dress up with a technical term.

The second reason for ready acceptance was probably that, in the name of helping someone to have a child, society seems to be willing to set aside any existing moral restraints and conventions. Perhaps in an underpopulated world, whose very existence is threatened by low birth rates, a case for artificial procreation might be made.

But it is hard to see why, in our world, where the problem of feckless and irresponsible male procreators is far more of a social crisis, society lets that one pass. One can well understand the urge, often desperate, to have a child. But it is less easy to understand an acceptance of the systematic downgrading of fatherhood brought about by the introduction of anonymous sperm donors. Or perhaps it was the case that fatherhood had already sunken to such a low state, and male irresponsibility was already so accepted, that no one saw a problem. It is as if everyone argued: Look, males have always been fathering children anonymously and irresponsibly; why not put this otherwise noxious trait to good use?

As a symbol of male irresponsibility—and a socially sanctioned symbol at that—one could hardly ask for anything better than artificial insemination with the sperm of anonymous donors. It raises male irresponsibility to the high level of a praised social institution, and it succeeds in getting males off the hook of fatherhood and parenthood in a strikingly effective and decisive way. The anonymity is an especially nice touch; no one will know who did what, and thus there can never be any moral accountability. That is the kind of world all of us have wished we could live in from time to time, especially in its sexual subdivision. From the perspective of the sperm donor, if the child's life turns out poorly, the donor will neither know about that nor inconveniently be called upon to provide help, fatherly help. Home free!

## IV. FEMINISM AND FATHERHOOD

As a movement, feminism has long had a dilemma on its hands. If women are to be free of the undue coercion and domination of males, they must establish their own independent sphere of activities and the necessary social and legal rights to protect that sphere. Women cannot and should not leave their fate in the hands of males, much less their reproductive fates. Meanwhile, feminists have also deplored feckless, irresponsible males who leave women in the lurch. Yet if males are to be encouraged to act more responsibly, to take seriously their duties to women and children, then they must be allowed to share the right to make decisions in those domains that bear on their activities and responsibilities. Males, moreover, have rights corresponding to their duties; they should be empowered to do that which their moral duties require of them.

For the most part, this dilemma has been resolved by the feminist movement in favor of stressing the independence of females from male control. This is evident in two important respects. First, in the abortion debate there has been a firm rejection of the claim that males should be either informed that a woman is considering an abortion or that the male should have a right to override her decision. The male should, in short, have neither a right to information nor choice about what happens to the conception.

Second, in its acceptance of single-parent procreation and motherhood, for both heterosexual and lesbian women, some branches of feminism have in effect declared fathers biologically irrelevant and socially unnecessary. Since this kind of motherhood requires, as a necessary condition, some male sperm (provided *in vitro* or *in vivo*), it has not been possible to dispense altogether with males. No such luck. But it has been possible to hold those males who assist such reproduction free of all responsibility for their action in providing the sperm. The only difference between the male who impregnates a woman in the course of sexual liaison and then disappears, and the man who is asked to disappear voluntarily after providing sperm, is that the latter kind of irresponsibility is, so to speak, licensed and legitimated. Indeed, it is treated as a kindly, beneficent action. The effect on the child is of course absolutely identical—an unknown, absent father.

Both of these moves seem understandable in the short run, but profoundly unhelpful to women in the long run. It is understandable why women would not want their abortion decision to depend upon male permission. They are the ones who will have to carry the child to term and nurture, as mothers, the child thereafter. It is no less understandable why some women want children without fathers. Some cannot find a male to marry but do not want to give up motherhood altogether; they view this as a course of necessity, a kind of lesser evil. Other women, for reasons of profound skepticism about males, or hostility toward them, simply want children apart from males altogether.

Please note that I said these motives are "understandable." I did not say they are justifiable. What is short-sighted about either of these choices is that, by their nullification of the moral obligations that ought to go with biological fatherhood, they contribute to the further infantilization of males, a phenomenon already well advanced in our society, and itself a long-standing source of harm for women.

If the obligations of males to take responsibility for the children they have procreated is sharply limited due to women deciding whether to grant males any rights, then males quickly get the message. That message is that the ordinary moral obligations that go with procreation are contingent and dispensable, not nearly as weighty as those of women. For even the most advanced feminists do not lightly allow women who have knowingly chosen to become mothers to jettison that obligation. Mothers are understood to be mothers forever, unlike fathers, who are understood to be fathers as long as no one has declared them free of responsibility. If you are a sperm donor, of course, that declaration can readily be had.

What social conditions are necessary to have the responsibilities of fatherhood taken seriously? The most obvious, it would seem, is a clear, powerful, and consistent social message to fathers: You are responsible for the lives of the children you procreate; you are always the father regardless of legal dispensations; only the gravest emergencies can relieve you of that obligation; you will be held liable if you fail in your duties; and, you will be given the necessary rights and prerogatives required to properly discharge your duties. Only recently has there been a concerted effort, long overdue, to require fathers to make good on child-support agreements. And only recently, and interestingly, has the importance of biological parenthood been sufficiently recognized to lower some of the barriers erected to keep adopted children from discovering the identity of their biological parents, including fathers.

Those feminists who believe that fathers should have no role in abortion decisions should reconsider that position or at least add some nuance. There are probably good reasons to not legally require that fathers be informed that the mother is considering an abortion; the possibilities of coercion and continuing stress thereafter are real and serious. But that is no reason to dispense with a *moral* requirement that the fathers be informed and their opinion requested if there are no overpowering reasons not to. The fetus that would be aborted is as much their doing as that of the mother, and the loss to the father can obviously be considerable. Acting as if the only serious consequences are for the woman is still another way of minimizing the importance of fatherhood.

Far too much is made of the fact that the woman actually carries the fetus. That does not make the child more hers than his, and in the lifetime span of procreation, childbearing, and child-rearing, the nine-month period of gestation is a minute portion of that span. Only very young parents who have not experienced the troubles of teenage children or an adult child's marital breakup could think of the woman's pregnancy as an especially significant or difficult time compared with other phases of parenthood.

Fathers, in short, have a moral right to know that they are fathers and to have a voice in decisions about the outcome of pregnancy. To deny males such a right is also to reject the very concept of paternal responsibility for one's procreative actions. The right to be a father cannot rest upon someone else's decision to grant such a right; that is no right at all. If the right to be a father is that poorly based, then there will be no better basis for upholding the moral obligations of fathers, or holding them accountable for their actions. I see no possibility of having it both ways. Society often asserts as a general principle that rights entail obligations. In this case, I am arguing the converse: If society wants obligations taken seriously, rights must be recognized.

The argument for a father's moral right to knowledge and choice does not entail a corresponding legal right to force a woman to bear a child against her will. There are a number of prudential and practical reasons not to require legal notification that a woman plans to have an abortion or to require the father's permission. Such a requirement, I suspect, would be both unworkable and probably destructive of many marital relationships. But as a moral norm, this requirement is perfectly appropriate. It puts moral pressure on women to see the need to inform fathers they are fathers, and to withhold such knowledge only when there are serious moral reasons to do so.

Women should, in general, want to do everything possible to encourage fathers to take their role and duties seriously. Women, and the children they bear, only lose if men are allowed to remain infantile and irresponsible. The attempt to encourage more responsible fatherhood and the sharing of childrearing duties while simultaneously promoting the total independence of women in their child-bearing decisions only sends a mixed message: Fathers should consider themselves responsible, but not too much; and they should share the choices and burdens of parenthood, but more the latter than the former; and all parents are created equal, but some are more equal than others.

I have mainly laid the emphasis so far on abortion decisions. But the same considerations apply when women, heterosexual or lesbian, make use of donated sperm deliberately to have a single-parent child. Women have been hurt throughout history by males who abandon their parental duties, leaving to women the task of raising the children. A sperm donor is doing exactly the same thing. The fact that he does it with social sanction does not change the outcome; one more male has been allowed to be a father without taking up the duties of fatherhood. Indeed, there is something symbolically destructive about using anonymous sperm donors to help women have children apart from a permanent marital relationship with the father.

For what action could more decisively declare the irrelevance of fatherhood than a specific effort to keep everyone ignorant? A male who would be a party to such an arrangement might well consider himself some kind of altruistic figure, helping women to get what they want. He would in reality be part of that grand old male tradition of fatherhood without tears, that wonderful fatherhood that permits all of the pleasures of procreation but none of its obligations. Women who use males in this way, allowing them to play once again that ancient role in a new guise, cannot fail to do harm both to women and parenthood.


## V. PARENTHOOD, FAMILIES, AND RELATIONSHIP

A great deal of fun is made these days of those old-fashioned families of the 1950s, especially the television versions, where the emphasis was placed on the family as a unit. They are spoofed in part because they failed to account for all of the families in those days that were simply not like that. Fair enough. They are derided as well because they often treated the women as empty-headed creatures good for nothing other than cleaning up after the kids and keeping father happy. And sometimes they are attacked because they did not present those fathers as strong leaders and role models for children. Rather, they portrayed fathers as weak and childish, capable of manipulation by wives and children.

But what the old-fashioned families saw clearly enough is that parenthood is a set of relationships, a complex web of rights, privileges, and duties as well as the more subtle interplay of morality in intimate relationships. Feminists have been prone to pose the problem of procreative rights as principally a female problem. Traditionalists have been wont to view fatherhood as a role of patriarchical hegemony. Both are wrong, however, because they fail to see the complexity of the relationship or to place the emphasis in the right place. Both mothers and fathers, as individual moral beings, have important roles as well as the rights and duties that go with those roles.

Those roles, most importantly, are conditioned by, and set in a context of, their mutuality. Each needs and is enriched by the role of the other. The obligations of the one are of benefit to the other; indeed, the mutuality of their obligations amplifies all of them. A mother can better be a mother if she has the active help of a father who takes his duties seriously. Likewise, the father will be a better father with the help of an equally serious mother. The child will, in turn, gain something from both of them, both individually and as a pair. It is important, therefore, that society return fatherhood to center stage not only for the sake of fathers, who will be forced to grow up, but also for mothers, who will benefit from a more mature notion of what fatherhood and parenthood are.

## References

1. Judith J. Thompson, *A Defense of Abortion*, 1 Phil. & Pub. Aff. 47, 65 (1971).
2. James L. Nelson, *Parental Obligations and the Ethics of Surrogacy: A Causal Perspective*, 5 Pub. Aff. Q. 49 (1991).
3. Mark S. Frankel, *Reproductive Technologies: Artificial Insemination*, 4 Encyclopedia of Bioethics 1439, 1444 (Warren T. Reich ed., 1978).
4. Daniel Wilder & Norma J. Wilder, *Turkey-baster Babies: The Demediealization of Artificial Insemination*, 69 Milbank Q. 5, 8 (1991).
5. See Frankel, *supra* note 3, at 1444.

# Index